Inflammatory
bowel disease

Simon Campbell MD MRCP

Specialist Registrar
Gastroenterology Unit
John Radcliffe Hospital,
Oxford,
UK

Simon Travis DPhil FRCP

Consultant Gastroenterologist
Gastroenterology Unit
John Radcliffe Hospital,
Oxford,
UK

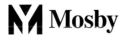 **Mosby**

Coventry University

MOSBY
An imprint of Elsevier Science Limited.

© 2004 Elsevier Science Ltd

The
Publisher's
policy is to use
**paper manufactured
from sustainable forests**

M Mosby is a registered trademark of Elsevier Science Limited.

ISBN 0-7234-3378-X

Cataloguing in Publication Data
Catalogue records for this book are available from the US Library of Congress and the British Library.

Note
Medical knowledge is constantly changing. As new information becomes available, changes in treatment, procedures, equipment and the use of drugs become necessary. The editors/authors/contributors and the publishers have taken care to ensure that the information given in this text is accurate and up to date. However, readers are strongly advised to confirm that the information, especially with regard to drug usage, complies with the latest legislation and standards of practice.

Printed in China.

Acknowledgements

We are grateful to friends and colleagues from the Gastroenterology Unit at Oxford for their comments, help and guidance on the manuscript. In particular, we would like to acknowledge Rupali Nicum for proof-reading the final version and giving comments from the primary care perspective. Acknowledgments and thanks should also go to Robert Edwards and Tuan Ho for their editorial support, and Roger Chapman, Helen Bungay and John Salmon for their help with illustrations throughout this text.

Simon Campbell and Simon Travis

Contents

Abbreviations

AS	ankylosing spondylitis
5-ASA	5-aminosalicylate
AZA	azathioprine
CD	Crohn's disease
CDA	Crohn's disease activity index
CRP	C-reactive protein
CsA	ciclosporin A
DXA	dual energy x-ray absorptiometry
EN	erythema nosodum
ERCP	endoscopic retrograde cholangiopancreatography
ESR	erythrocyte sedimentation rate
FBC	full blood count
Hb	haemoglobin
HBI	Harvey-Bradshaw index
HLA	human leukocyte antigen
IBD	inflammatory bowel diseases
IFX	infliximab
LFT	liver function test
MP	mercaptopurine
MR	magnetic resonance
MTX	methotrexate
NNT	number needed to treat
NSAID	non-steroidal anti-inflammtory drug
PG	pyoderma grangrenosum
PSC	primary sclerosing cholangitis
TPMT	thiopurine methyl transferase
UC	ulcerative colitis
U&Es	urea and electrolytes

Introduction and background

Epidemiology

There is an abundance of good data on the incidence of ulcerative colitis (UC) and Crohn's disease (CD).[1] In both conditions, there is a similar incidence between the sexes, despite a slight preponderance of males with UC and females with CD.[2] Both conditions become more common with increasing latitude from the equator for reasons that are unclear. Inflammatory bowel disease (IBD) is more common in countries such as Iceland, Scandinavia and North America compared with countries such as Greece, southern Spain or Italy, as illustrated in Table 1.

About 240,000 people are affected by IBD in the UK, where the annual incidence of UC ranges from seven to 22 new cases per 100,000 per year,[3] with no apparent increase in incidence recently. Asian immigrants have a much higher incidence than their counterparts in the sub-continent. The prevalence is 90–170 per 100,000 people (twice as common as CD), but studies from primary care on hospital-diagnosed cases report up to 268 per 100,000.

Table 1. Incidence rates for ulcerative colitis and Crohn's disease in countries from around the world*		
	Ulcerative colitis	**Crohn's disease**
Northern centres	**Incidence rates per 100,000**	
Iceland	24.3	8.2
Norway	15.6	6.9
Netherlands	13.1	7.7
Southern Centres	**Incidence rates per 100,000**	
Italy	10.0	3.2
Spain	7.0	4.8
Sicily	8.5	5.8

*Data taken from Shivananda S, Lennard-Jones J, Logan R et al. Incidence of inflammatory bowel disease across Europe: is there a difference between north and south? Results of the European Collaborative Study on Inflammatory Bowel Disease (EC-IBD). Gut 1996;**39**:690–7.

For CD, the incidence is around four to 11 per 100,000.[4;5] The prevalence of CD is 70–100 per 100,000 population, but studies from primary care on hospital-diagnosed cases report a higher prevalence (156/100,000). The incidence of CD has doubled since 1950 and increased until 1990, but appears stable in northern Europe.[6-8] The prevalence of IBD does not differ markedly between race, sex or social class in Europe, although is more common among Jews in the USA.

Aetiology and pathogenesis

The aetiologies of both UC and CD remain unknown. The consensus is that both diseases are a response to environmental triggers (infection, drugs or other agents) in genetically susceptible individuals.[8] The genetic component is stronger in CD than in UC. Smoking increases the risk of CD but decreases the risk of UC through unknown mechanisms.

Concepts

Theories and evidence for pathogenetic mechanisms are too complex to be considered in a *Rapid Reference* guide. The broad areas examined are epidemiology, the gut: environmental interface, and the inflammatory process and genetics of each disease. Epidemiological studies have considered diet, drug and vaccination history, seasonal variation, water supply and social circumstances. Smoking is not causative but is the most consistently related environmental factor.

Bacteria, epithelium and mucosal inflammation

The gut:environmental interface includes work on luminal bacteria, biofilms, the epithelial glycocalyx and mucus, epithelial barrier function, epithelial remodelling and immune–epithelial interactions. The implications for therapy are that antibiotics, or probiotics, and factors such as epidermal growth factor that promote epithelial repair may have a role in management. The inflammatory process has been examined through cell-signalling pathways, cytokine profiles, eicosanoids and other inflammatory mediators, lymphocyte trafficking, cell-surface molecules, interactions between stromal and immune cells, and neuroimmune communication. It is these processes that are the main target of aminosalicylates, corticosteroids, immunomodulators and new biological agents.

Genetic factors

Twin studies illustrate the genetic component, because 44% of monozygotic pairs have CD together[9] (*see Inflammatory bowel diseases in pregnancy, children and adolescents*). Genetics have adopted a candidate-gene approach, genome-wide screening through microsatellite markers and, most recently, studies on functional gene expression. Mutations of one gene (CARD15/NOD2), located on chromosome 16,[10] have been associated with small intestinal CD in Caucasian (but not Oriental) populations. Two other genes have recently been identified and the existence of others is strongly suggested by replicated linkage to a number of chromosomes.[11] The implications are that it may be possible to predict the pattern of disease from a patient's genotype and tailor treatment to the individual, although this has yet to be realized.

Clinical presentation

Presentation of ulcerative colitis

The cardinal symptom of UC is bloody diarrhoea.[12] Associated symptoms of colicky abdominal pain, urgency or tenesmus may be present. UC is a potentially severe disease that used to carry a high mortality and major morbidity. With modern medical and surgical management, the disease has now a slight excess of mortality in the first year after diagnosis, but no subsequent difference from the normal population (*see Prognosis*). However, a severe attack of UC is still a potentially life-threatening illness.

Presentation of Crohn's disease

Symptoms of CD are more heterogeneous, but typically include abdominal pain, diarrhoea and weight loss.[12] Systemic symptoms of malaise, anorexia or fever are more common with CD than UC. CD may cause intestinal obstruction owing to strictures, fistulae (often perianal) or abscesses. Diarrhoea is not often bloody, even in those with colonic disease, because inflammation in CD is transmural rather than mucosal.

Referral pathway

As a rule, any patient with diarrhoea that persists for more than 2 weeks merits specialist referral, especially if associated with weight loss. The difference between bloody diarrhoea and a change in bowel habit with rectal bleeding is relevant. The former condition should be referred to a gastro-enterologist, and the latter to a colorectal surgeon. Patients with bloody diarrhoea and a frequency greater than six times a day should be referred urgently by telephone. (*See* Table 2 for referral pathway.)

Table 2. Referral pathways for patients with diarrhoea		
Clinical situation	**Route of referral**	**Investigations before referral**
Diarrhoea > 2 weeks without nocturnal symptoms	Gastroenterology; routine	Stool C&S; FBC; CRP; EMA; U&Es; LFTs
Diarrhoea > 2 weeks with nocturnal frequency or weight loss	Gastroenterology; urgent	Stool C&S; FBC; CRP; EMA; U&Es; LFTs; TFTs
Bloody diarrhoea < 6 times/day	Gastroenterology; urgent or telephone gastroenterologist if found to be anaemic	Stool C&S; FBC; CRP; U&Es; LFTs; stool *C. difficile* toxin assay if antibiotics or proton-pump inhibitor in past 2 months
Bloody diarrhoea > 6 times/day with tachycardia, fever or anaemia	Arrange admission or telephone gastroenterologist	FBC; CRP; stool C&S and *C. difficile* toxin assay; document pulse rate and temperature
Increased bowel frequency with rectal bleeding	Colorectal surgery; urgent	FBC; CRP; LFTs

C&S = culture and sensitivity; FBC = full blood count; CRP = C-reactive protein;
EMA = endomysial antibody (in case of coeliac disease);
U&Es = urea and electrolytes (hypokalaemia suggests severe diarrhoea);
LFTs = liver function tests; TFTs = thyroid function tests

Diagnosis and investigations

General

The diagnosis of UC or CD is established by clinical evaluation and a combination of biochemical, endoscopic, radiological and histological investigations, as well as those based on nuclear medicine. Brief details are given because it is assumed that the diagnosis is established at a specialist hospital clinic.

Criteria for ulcerative colitis

In the case of UC, the diagnosis should be made on the basis of clinical suspicion supported by appropriate macroscopic findings on sigmoidoscopy or colonoscopy, typical histological findings on biopsy, and negative stool examinations for infectious agents.

Criteria for Crohn's disease

For CD, the diagnosis depends on demonstrating focal, asymmetric and often granulomatous inflammation, but the investigations selected vary according to the presenting manifestations, physical findings and complications.

Indeterminate colitis

When the type of colitis cannot be defined confidently as either UC or CD, the term "indeterminate colitis" is appropriate.[9] This occurs in 7–10% of patients, usually because the patient's clinical features (e.g. non-bloody diarrhoea) do not match the endoscopic appearance (e.g. continuous mucosal inflammation), and histology is non-specific (e.g. absence of granulomas). Indeterminate colitis usually follows the pattern of UC, but its principal importance is in decision-making for the small proportion of patients who need an ileo-anal pouch (*see Surgical therapy in inflammatory bowel diseases*).

Laboratory investigations
All patients with active disease
For all new patients and those who relapse, laboratory investigations should include full blood count (FBC), urea and electrolytes (U&Es), liver function tests (LFTs) and erythrocyte sedimentation rate (ESR) or C-reactive protein (CRP), as well as microbiological testing for infectious diarrhoea including *Clostridium difficile* toxin. Additional tests for ova, cysts and parasites are appropriate for patients who have travelled abroad. Abdominal radiography is essential in the initial assessment of patients with suspected severe IBD: it excludes colonic dilatation and may help assess disease extent in UC or identify proximal constipation. In CD, abdominal radiography may give an impression of a mass in the right iliac fossa, or show evidence of small bowel dilatation.

Other investigations
Imaging the colon
For mild to moderate disease, colonoscopy is usually preferable to flexible sigmoidoscopy, because the extent of disease can be assessed, but in moderate to severe disease there is a higher risk of bowel perforation and flexible sigmoidoscopy is safer. For suspected CD, colonoscopy to the terminal ileum and small bowel barium studies to define extent and site of disease are appropriate. A terminal ileal biopsy performed at colonoscopy documents the extent of examination, and may find microscopic evidence of CD. Other conditions (including tuberculosis, Behcet's syndrome, lymphoma, vasculitis) may also cause ileal disease. Double-contrast barium enema is inferior to colonoscopy, because it does not allow mucosal biopsy and may underestimate the extent of disease.

Small-bowel imaging
Small bowel enema (*via* nasojejunal intubation) or barium follow-through (oral barium) remains the procedure of choice

for diagnosing small intestinal CD. The role of capsule endoscopy is at present unclear. White cell scanning is a safe non-invasive investigation, but lacks specificity. Ultrasound in skilled hands is a sensitive and non-invasive way of identifying thickened small bowel loops in CD, and may identify abscesses or free fluid in the peritoneum.

Imaging for complications
Computed tomography scanning and magnetic resonance (MR) imaging, especially of the perineum, help evaluate activity and complications of disease. Laparoscopy may be necessary in selected patients, especially where the differential diagnosis of intestinal tuberculosis is being considered.

Disease extent

After the diagnosis of UC or CD has been confirmed, the disease extent should be defined because it determines the best route for therapy. For UC, the extent is defined as the proximal margin of macroscopic inflammation because this is most clearly related to the risk of complications, including dilatation and cancer. The implications of limited macroscopic disease with extensive microscopic inflammation remain unclear. For CD, both small bowel and colon should be assessed.

Disease severity

Precise framework

For each individual with UC or CD, the activity, extent and pattern of disease need to be defined. The activity describes the severity at a point in time, the extent refers to the distribution of disease (established at diagnosis; *see* earlier), while the pattern describes the frequency of relapse and duration of remission (*see* later). These factors are the basis for making therapeutic decisions and affect the prognosis, so they should be highlighted in clinical notes for individual patients.

Severity of ulcerative colitis

For UC, the severity is most simply assessed by the Truelove and Witts' criteria (Table 3).[10] Its real value is in everyday clinical practice, because it defines an approach to management, and it is so easy to underestimate the severity of disease. It cannot be used for following the pattern of disease, which is more relevant to clinical trials, and other indices (e.g. the Simple Clinical Colitis Index) are designed for this.[11,14]

Severity of Crohn's disease

For CD, severity is more difficult to assess.[15] Most clinicians evaluate symptom severity subjectively in combination with CRP measurement, which usually confirms active inflammation as a cause of symptoms. The Crohn's disease activity index (CDAI; Table 4) is a research tool by virtue of its complexity and is too cumbersome to use in everyday clinical practice, although it is the standard in most clinical trials. The Harvey-Bradshaw index (HBI; Table 5) is an abbreviated score that is potentially useful for clinical practice and correlates well with the CDAI.[12] Activity indices are becoming more important, because they are being advocated as a gating or audit system for expensive new biological therapy such as infliximab (IFX). For this purpose, the HBI is a more useful tool.

Table 3. Truelove and Witts' criteria for severity of ulcerative colitis*			
	Mild	**Moderate**	**Severe**
Bloody stool frequency	< 4 times/day	In-between mild and severe	> 6 times/day
Pulse rate	Normal		> 90 bpm
Temperature	Normal		> 37.8°C
Haemoglobin	Normal		< 10.5 g/dl
ESR	Normal		> 30 mm/hr

*Only one criterion in addition to stool frequency defines severe disease
ESR = erythrocyte sedimentation rate

Table 4. Crohn's disease activity index (CDAI)

Days 1–7 prospective diary	Sum	x (factor)	Score
Number liquid/very soft stools	–	2	–
Abdominal pain rating (0 = none; 1 = mild; 2 = moderate; 3 = severe)	–	5	–
General well-being (0 = generally well; 1 = slightly under par; 2 = poor; 3 = very poor; 4 = terrible)	–	7	–
Number of extra-intestinal manifestations (arthritis/arthralgia; iritis/anterior uveitis; erythema nodosum/pyoderma gangrenosum; anal fissure; fistula; fever > 37.0 °C in past week)	–	20	–
Taking antidiarrhoeals (no = 0; yes = 30)	–	1	–
Abdominal mass (0 = none; 20 = questionable; 50 = definite)	–	1	–
Haematocrit (males 47-haematocrit; females 42-haematocrit)	–	6	–
Body weight (% below standard weight for height – add if below, subtract if overweight)	–	1	–
Total = CDAI*	–		–

*CDAI < 150 = remission; CDAI 150–300 = moderately active; CDAI > 300 = severe disease

Table 5. Harvey-Bradshaw index for Crohn's disease activity*

	Parameter	Score
A	General well-being	0 = very well; 1 = slightly below par; 2 = poor; 3 = very poor; 4 = terrible
B	Abdominal pain	0 = none; 1 = mild; 2 = moderate; 3 = severe
C	Number of liquid stools per day	
D	Abdominal mass	0 = none; 1 = dubious; 2 = definite; 3 = definite and tender
E	Extra-intestinal complications	Score 1 for each of arthralgia, uveitis, erythema nodosum, aphthous ulcers, pyoderma gangrenosum, anal fissure, new fistula, abscess

*Score < 5 = remission; score 5–9 = moderate disease; score > 9 = severe disease

Pattern of disease

Defining different patterns

The clinical course of UC is marked by exacerbations and remission. There are broadly three patterns: infrequent relapse (< once/year), frequent relapse (> once/year) and, for a few, continuous active disease.

Pattern of ulcerative colitis

For UC, about 50% of patients have a relapse in any year. An appreciable minority has frequently relapsing or chronic, continuous disease and, overall, 20–30% of patients with pancolitis come to colectomy.

Pattern of Crohn's disease

The clinical course of CD is also characterized by exacerbations and remission. In CD, surgery is not curative and management is directed to minimizing the impact of disease. At least 50% of patients require surgical treatment in the first 10 years of disease and approximately 70–80% will require surgery within their lifetime.

The pattern and prognosis (*see Prognosis*) are important considerations when discussing the implications for insurance, and detailed advice is published or available from the National Association for Colitis and Crohn's (NACC; website: www.nacc.org.uk; tel.: 01727 820038).

Clinical problem: first presentation of bloody diarrhoea

The following factors should be addressed in the following order.

History: acute or chronic?

Acute (< 2 weeks) duration suggests infection (e.g. *Campylobacter* sp., *E. coli* 0157:H7 or *Shigella* sp., but not *Salmonella* sp.), especially if there have been contacts with someone having a similar history or there is associated vomiting. Longer (> 2 weeks) but not definitive duration, lack of contacts or travel abroad, or a family history of IBD are markers that would favour IBD.

Clinical examination

Tachycardia, pyrexia or dehydration are markers of severity (Table 3), and indicate the need for telephone referral to a hospital for admission. Urgent out-patient assessment is otherwise appropriate if there is no systemic disturbance.

Investigations

Stool should be sent for culture. If the patient has had antibiotics within the previous 6 weeks, then a specific request should be made for *C. difficile* toxin assay. The FBC, CRP, U&Es and albumin should be performed. A normal CRP does not exclude UC or CD, but indicates that it is only mildly active if present or limited in extent. An abdominal radiograph is appropriate, if there is systemic upset, to exclude toxic dilatation.

Other investigations

The quickest way to diagnose or exclude UC is by rectal examination and rigid sigmoidoscopy, which should always be performed unless there are immediate plans to perform a flexible sigmoidoscopy. The rectal mucosa is always abnormal in UC. Infective colitis occasionally looks similar to UC in the early stages, but UC should always be suspected until proven otherwise. If the rectal mucosa is normal, the possibilities are Crohn's colitis (an unusual cause of bloody diarrhoea), sigmoid carcinoma (even less common; a rectal carcinoma should have been detected), or haemorrhoids and another cause of diarrhoea.

Treatment

When a diagnosis of infective colitis is certain, no treatment is necessary unless there is systemic upset (fever, tachycardia and dehydration). Ciprofloxacin 500 mg twice daily for 5 days is then reasonable. Microbiologists still prefer to wait for a positive stool culture, but the clinical situation does not always allow this. When the diagnosis is clearly UC, steroids are appropriate according to severity (*see* Table 7 in section *Medical therapy*). When there is diagnostic doubt, it is safest to treat **both** conditions (i.e. with steroids and antibiotics, pending the results of investigation) rather than leave potential UC untreated.

Extra-intestinal manifestations in inflammatory bowel diseases

Introduction

Extra-intestinal manifestations affect the joints, skin, eyes and hepatobiliary system. They usually correlate with colonic disease (Crohn's colitis or UC) and are less common when CD is confined to the small bowel.[13] They affect a minority of patients (about 15% of all cases of IBD), but cause appreciable morbidity.

Relation to pattern of disease

In contrast to acute manifestations (erythema nodosum, arthropathy or ophthalmic conditions), the course of more chronic disorders (hepatobiliary complications, ankylosing spondylitis [AS]) is generally unrelated to IBD disease activity.

Ophthalmic conditions

Episcleritis

Episcleritis (Figure 1) is the most common ocular feature of IBD. It presents with redness and discomfort, but may very rarely cause superficial ulceration of the sclera and almost always resolves with treatment of the active colitis.

Iritis (anterior uveitis)

Iritis, or anterior and uveitis (Figure 2), occurs less frequently. A reported prevalence of 2–3% appears to be an overestimate. Patients with UC or CD are equally affected, although some studies suggest that the rate of iritis/anterior uveitis is higher in CD.[14-16] Pain can precede redness, but the classic presentation is a decreased visual acuity with a painful red eye. Urgent referral to an ophthalmologist is essential, because delay in treatment can cause permanent damage. Topical steroids and mydriatics are effective in conjunction with treatment of the active colitis.

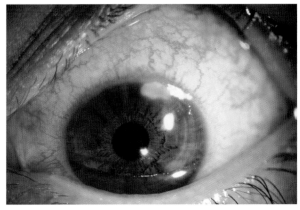

Figure 1. Episcleritis.

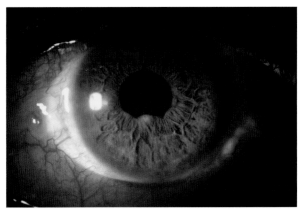

Figure 2. Iritis (anterior uveitis).

Cutaneous manifestations

Erythema nodosum

Erythema nodosum (EN) is the most common cutaneous manifestation of IBD. It presents as tender, raised, red lesions about the size of a 50-pence coin, which are classically seen on the shins. EN is usually associated with active IBD, affecting predominantly women with Crohn's colitis (68% CD *vs* 32%UC), and its reported prevalence varies between

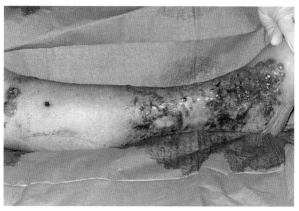

Figure 3. Pyoderma grangrenosum affecting the lower limbs.

2 and 15%.[16-18] Recognition and treatment of the underlying active IBD will result in the regression of this condition.

Pyoderma grangrenosum

Pyoderma grangrenosum (PG) is less common but, like EN, is part of the spectrum of acute neutrophilic dermatoses and also predominantly affects women with Crohn's colitis. PG lesions are usually single and affect points of contact – often the lower limbs (Figure 3), back or peristomal region – and are characterized by deep ulcers with purple edges and a purulent sterile discharge. Management of PG can be difficult because treatment of active IBD may be insufficient, and the condition may recur after colectomy. Traditionally, high doses of steroids are used but, like many extra-intestinal manifestations, PG usually responds extremely well to IFX.[19] Specialist advice is appropriate.

Rheumatological conditions

Spectrum

There are four main rheumatological disorders associated with IBD: sacroiliitis, AS, a pauciarticular large joint arthropathy and a polyarticular small joint arthropathy.[20] Osteoarthritis and rheumatoid arthritis are seen at frequencies similar to that of the general population, although those who have IBD and psoriasis are more likely to develop psoriatic arthropathy. Osteoporosis is covered in section *Complications of inflammatory bowel diseases*.

Sacroiliitis

Sacroiliitis is the most common condition, with a reported prevalence up to 18%, although this condition may remain asymptomatic. Despite being a feature of AS, sacroiliitis usually occurs in isolation and, unlike AS, is unrelated to human leukocyte antigen (HLA) status.[21;22]

Clinical features

When symptomatic, sacroiliitis causes low-back pain and morning stiffness (similar to AS), but no peripheral joint symptoms. Symptoms are often worse during active disease. Pressure on the sacroiliac joints on clinical examination causes pain. Sclerosis of the sacroiliac joints on x-ray is diagnostic (Figure 4), although MR scanning is more sensitive.

Treatment

Simple analgesics are usually sufficient until the joints fuse.

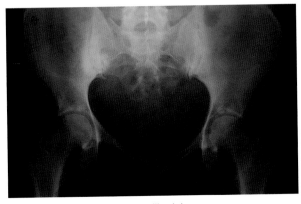

Figure 4. Sclerosis of the sacroiliac joints on x-ray.

Ankylosing spondylitis

About 2–7% of IBD patients have AS, with no difference between UC and CD.[23;24] Some patients have back pain or arthralgia without a formal diagnosis of AS.

Clinical symptoms

Symptoms of early morning stiffness and low-back pain are typical. There is limited movement of the lumbar lordosis on forward flexion. Pain may be severe and radiate into the abdomen. Peripheral joints may be affected. The clinical course of AS is independent of the IBD. A combination of clinical and radiological markers are used in the diagnosis of AS. Radiological evidence of sacroiliitis and a positive HLA-B27 are diagnostic, although a bone scan or MR scan is more sensitive for detecting AS.

Treatment

Physiotherapy and non-steroidal anti-inflammatory drug (NSAID) therapy are central to the management of AS. Both standard NSAIDs and cyclooxygenase-2 (COX-2) inhibitors have the potential for exacerbating colitis but, if the clinical symptoms cannot be controlled with simple analgesics, the risk has to be taken. Many people can manage NSAIDs, but they should not be prescribed without warning the patient that their colitis may deteriorate. Sulfasalazine is theoretically more appropriate than mesalazine, because of its potential arthropathy-modifying effect. In practice, other immuno-modulators (such as methotrexate [MTX]) are often necessary. IFX gives very good symptom relief, but it is unclear whether it alters the pattern of AS, which progresses independently of the pattern of IBD and may lead to appreciable debility.

Pauciarticular, large joint arthropathy

This is an asymmetrical, sero-negative arthropathy that parallels disease activity.[20]

Clinical symptoms

Arthropathy characteristically affects a hip, knee or ankle. The pattern is established early in the course of IBD, and it may predate intestinal symptoms. Because it is transient and non-destructive, the point prevalence has been reported as low as 0.8%.[25]

Treatment

This condition responds to treatment of the active colitis, and does not lead to deformity. As for AS, sulfasalazine is a rational maintenance therapy.

Polyarticular, small joint arthropathy

Clinical symptoms

In contrast to the previous condition, this arthropathy is unrelated to disease activity.[24] The distinction between the two arthropathies is reflected in different genetic associations.[25;26] The arthropathy is symmetrical, characteristically affecting the finger joints. It is more common and more troublesome than the pauciarticular form, because pain persists.

Treatment

Analgesics (with the same caveats about NSAIDs; *see* earlier) and physiotherapy are appropriate. Disease-modifying therapy does not have an appreciable impact, but deformity does not develop.

Hepatobiliary disease

Spectrum

There are three main hepatobiliary problems that can occur in IBD: intrinsic liver disease, primary sclerosing cholangitis (PSC) and cholelithiasis. At least 10% of IBD patients will develop deranged LFTs at some point in their disease course. The diagnosis and management of the underlying cause are important. Table 6 summarizes the usual patterns of deranged LFTs in IBD.

Table 6. Usual patterns of abnormal liver function tests in inflammatory bowel diseases

Condition	ALT or AST	ALP	Bilirubin	PT	Comments
Acute relapse of ulcerative colitis or Crohn's disease	x 1–2	x 1–1.5	N	N	Resolves with remission
Sulfasalazine hepatotoxicity	x 2–10	x 1.5–3	N–x 10	N	2–3 weeks after starting; no chronic disease
Azathioprine hepatotoxicity	x 2–10	x 1.5–3	N–x 10	N	2–3 weeks after starting; no chronic disease
Primary sclerosing cholangitis	N	x 2–10	N–x 20	N	Usually male with quiescent pancolitis; progression over years
Common bile duct stones	x 1–2	x 2–5	x 2–> 10	N	Sudden onset with pain
Other causes	Any	Any	Any	N– x 2	Check alcohol history, other drugs, travel, HBV and HCV, auto-antibodies – see Figure 6

ALT = alanine transaminase; AST = aspartate transaminase; PT = prothrombin time; x 1–2 = normal to 2-fold elevation; N = usually normal; HBV = hepatitis B virus; HCV = hepatitis C virus

Intrinsic liver disease

Deranged LFTs during an acute relapse are common, and do not merit investigation unless enzymes remain persistently abnormal when in remission for more than 2 months (*see Clinical problem: dealing with deranged liver function tests in inflammatory bowel diseases*).

Causes

Steatosis is the likely cause and does not progress. Other causes (alcohol, hepatitis B or C, autoimmune hepatitis and

PSC) should be considered if LFTs remain abnormal after treatment of active disease. Autoimmune hepatitis is associated with UC more commonly than CD. It is recognised by positive autoantibodies (anti-smooth muscle and anti-nuclear antibodies) and diagnosed by liver biopsy. Drugs should always be considered as a potential cause of deranged LFTs. The rare hepatotoxicity associated with sulfasalazine or azathioprine (AZA) is, however, characterized by an acute illness with an elevated aspartate aminotransferase level 2–3 weeks after starting therapy. Neither agent causes chronic liver disease when used, and tolerated, for maintenance therapy.

Investigations
Biopsy is usually only appropriate if the aspartate aminotransferase level remains more than double (*see also Immunomodulotherapy – Methotrexate; Side effects*). If the alkaline phosphatase level is also elevated, an overlap syndrome between PSC and autoimmune hepatitis should be considered; both biopsy and endoscopic retrograde cholangiopancreatography (ERCP) should be performed. Specialist management is appropriate. In contrast to PSC, granulomatous hepatitis is more common in CD than UC. Typically, LFTs are cholestatic (i.e. alanine phosphatase disproportionately elevated compared with aspartate aminotransferase or alanine transferase).[27-29]

Primary sclerosing cholangitis
PSC is a chronic, progressive cholestatic liver disease characterized by continuing inflammation, necrosis, and obliteration of intrahepatic and extrahepatic bile ducts.

Clinical symptoms
The male:female ratio for PSC is 2:1; this condition is more common in UC (prevalence 2–4%) and often affects patients with quiescent pancolitis.[30;31] Diagnosis is most often made after an elevated alkaline phosphatase level is detected

coincidentally on routine blood testing, in advance of symptoms (*see* later). The pathognomonic histological feature is an onion-skin appearance of concentric rings of connective tissue obliterating bile-duct canaliculi. Over time, these lesions cause bile-duct strictures with areas of intrahepatic bile-duct dilatation, causing a beaded appearance (Figure 5). ERCP remains the "gold standard" for diagnosis but is invasive, potentially introduces infection into the biliary tree and is becoming unnecessary if magnetic resonance cholangiography shows a characteristic appearance.

Treatment
There is currently no medical treatment that affects the course of the disease. Ursodeoxycholic acid is, however, widely used

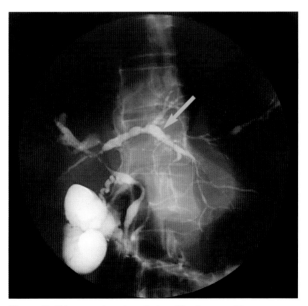

Figure 5. Primary sclerosing cholangitis diagnosed by endoscopic retrograde cholangiopancreatography (ERCP): bile-duct strictures, with areas of intrahepatic bile-duct dilatation, cause a beaded appearance (arrow).

to treat PSC because it improves the results of biochemical LFTs[32] and is safe. It does not alter histological progression. Cholestasis progresses at a variable rate, resulting in cirrhosis and portal hypertension.

Outcome
Median survival is 12 years after diagnosis, although this is changing with liver transplantation. The major clinical issues for patients with PSC are the development of cholangio-carcinoma (up to 30% patients) and a higher incidence of colorectal neoplasia. Sudden worsening of cholestasis or the development of jaundice in a patient with PSC should raise the possibility of a cholangiocarcinoma. The higher risk of colorectal cancer is an indication for annual surveillance colonoscopy after disease of 10 years' duration.

Cholelithiasis

Gallstones are more common in patients with CD, because ileal disease or resection interrupts the enterohepatic circulation of bile acids, resulting in lithogenic bile. The clinical message is that gallstones should be considered as a cause of pain in patients with CD, rather than assuming that pain is due to active intestinal disease.

Clinical problem: dealing with deranged liver function tests in inflammatory bowel diseases

Initial assessment

The prevalence of deranged LFTs is about 10%. The history should be reviewed, disease activity assessed and a decision then made about investigation. Key components of the history include symptoms of itching (due to the cholestasis of PSC), pain (consider common bile-duct calculi), drugs (duration and dose), alcohol intake and features of active disease (such as stool frequency).

Period of observation

If the disease is active, deranged LFTs are usually attributable to the systemic illness, sepsis or poor nutrition, and simply need to be rechecked every 1–2 weeks during treatment and then after 6–8 weeks in remission to ensure that they return to normal.

Further investigation

If abnormal LFTs persist during remission, further blood tests should be performed, including hepatitis B and C serology, autoantibodies, immunoglobulins and prothrombin time. An ultrasound should be requested to look for gallstones, biliary dilatation or focal lesions, although non-specific variations in hepatic echogenicity are commonly reported. Assuming no focal pathology is identified, a liver biopsy should be performed, whether there is a predominant elevation of transaminases or alkaline phosphatase, or a mixed pattern. If cholestasis is present (alkaline phosphatase more than double), magnetic resonance cholangiography, if available, is appropriate before ERCP to identify PSC. Figure 6 illustrates an algorithm for investigating abnormal LFTs.

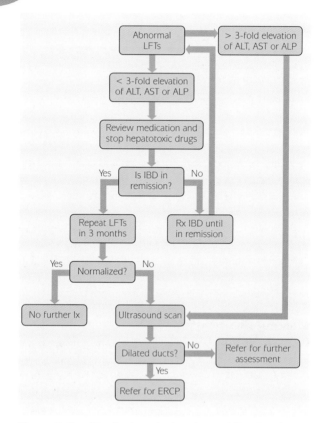

Figure 6. Algorithm for investigating abnormal liver function tests (LFTs = liver function tests; ALT = alanine aminotransferase ; AST = aspartate amnitransferase ; ALP = alkaline phosphatase ; IBD = inflammatory bowel disease ; Rx = treatment; Ix = investigation; ERCP = endoscopic retrograde cholangiopancreatography).

Medical therapy

Introduction

Corticosteroids and 5-aminosalicylate (5-ASA) drugs have remained the cornerstone of medical therapy for both UC and CD for almost 40 years. We are on the threshold of new biological therapy[33] and major changes can be expected in the next 5 years. Nevertheless, most new agents are designed to induce remission, with few expected to make the transition to maintenance therapy to prevent relapse. In contrast, the long-established AZA or 6-mercaptopurine (MP) are increasingly used for maintaining remission in frequently relapsing, steroid-refractory or steroid-resistant UC and CD. Other immunomodulators have specific roles, including ciclosporin A (CsA) for severe UC and MTX for chronic active CD.

Therapeutic strategy

For both UC and CD, the therapeutic strategy should first involve induction of remission and then maintenance therapy to reduce the risk of relapse. It is important that the patient understands this two-phase approach, because agents that induce remission are frequently less effective at maintaining remission, and *vice versa*. Therapeutic decisions also depend on disease **activity, extent** (or location) and **pattern** (*see Introduction and background – Disease extent; Disease severity; Pattern of disease*). Finally, monitoring is necessary to detect and treat complications.

Ulcerative colitis

Active disease should be assessed objectively (*see Introduction and Background – Disease severity*) and treated decisively according to extent. Disease extent can broadly be divided into distal and more extensive disease (Figure 7). Topical management is the appropriate initial therapy for active distal disease. If remission (stool frequency ≤ 3/day

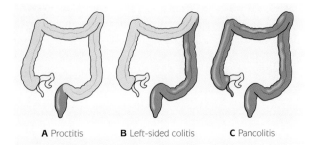

A Proctitis   **B** Left-sided colitis   **C** Pancolitis

Figure 7. Extent of bowel involvement in different degrees of ulcerative colitis: (A) ulcerative protitis (involvement limited to the rectum); (B) distal or left-sided colitis (inflammation extends 40 cm from the rectum); (C) pancolitis (colonic inflammation beyond the splenic flexure).

without visible blood) is not achieved within 2 weeks, then oral steroids are generally appropriate because high-dose 5-ASA (4 g/day) acts more slowly and is less effective. For those with active, extensive disease, oral steroids are the first line of treatment in the UK and Europe. Once remission is achieved, maintenance therapy with a 5-ASA is appropriate; if, however, the patient has required two or more courses of steroids within 12 months, then immunomodulators should be introduced. Colectomy improves the quality of life for refractory disease, but is only necessary in a minority of patients (< 10% of those with distal and < 30% of those with extensive disease). Maintenance therapy is generally continued long-term, although it is reasonable to discuss stopping therapy for those patients who have been in remission for more than 2 years. Patients who then relapse within a few months usually benefit from life-long therapy. The frequency of monitoring depends on the pattern and extent of disease. Indications for surveillance colonoscopy and the influence of 5-ASA on reducing the risk of colorectal cancer are discussed later in this section.

Crohn's disease

The severity of CD is more difficult to assess than UC (*see Introduction and Background – Disease severity*).

The general principles are to consider the site (ileal, ileocolic, colonic or others), pattern (inflammatory, structuring or fistulating) and activity of the disease before treatment decisions are made. Decisive treatment with a short (6–8 weeks) course of steroids remains most appropriate for many patients with active disease. However, an alternative explanation for symptoms other than active disease should be considered (such as bacterial overgrowth, bile salt malabsorption, dysmotility or gallstones) and disease activity confirmed, usually by CRP or ESR, before starting steroids. Furthermore, alternatives to steroids should be discussed with the patient. Alternatives to steroids are especially appropriate if symptoms are mild and not interfering with lifestyle (consider high-dose 5-ASA or antibiotics), or if steroids have been used within the past 6 months (AZA is indicated as a steroid-sparing agent). Other options include budesonide (for ileal disease), nutritional therapy (for continuous symptoms in adults or for adolescents) or surgery (for fistulating disease or obstructive symptoms). Preventing relapse is often more difficult than for UC. Maintenance therapy with 5-ASA is less effective, and the most important dictum is that patients who smoke should be advised, and helped, to stop.

5-Aminosalicylates

These include mesalazine, or 5-ASA (also called "mesalamine" in the USA).

Choice and mechanism

Various formulations are used to deliver millimolar concentrations to the gut lumen. 5-ASA is available as oral tablets, sachets or suspension, liquid or foam enemas, or suppositories. They act topically by a variety of mechanisms to moderate the release of inflammatory mediators and reactive oxygen species. Oral forms include:

- pH-dependent release/resin-coated (Asacol®, Salofalk® or Ipocol®)
- time-controlled release (Pentasa®)

- delivery by carrier molecules, with release of 5-ASA after splitting by bacterial enzymes in the large intestine (sulfasalazine [Salazopyrin®], olsalazine [Dipentum®], balsalazide [Colazide®]).

Maintenance of remission

The main role for 5-ASA is maintenance of remission in UC. Individual 5-ASA derivatives all show comparable efficacy to sulfasalazine, but in a meta-analysis the parent compound had a modest therapeutic advantage for maintaining remission (odds ratio 1.29; confidence interval 1.08–1.57).[34] The choice probably matters since delivery system is best matched to the site of disease. Azo-bonded compounds may be better for distal disease, which predominates in UC, and olsalazine was found to be better than Asacol[35] in one of very few direct comparisons between 5-ASA derivatives. Other considerations in the choice of 5-ASA are tolerability (mesalazine is tolerated by 80% of those unable to tolerate sulfasalazine), dose schedule (twice-daily dosing is associated with better compliance) and cost.[36] Maintenance therapy with all 5-ASA drugs probably reduces the risk of colorectal cancer by 75% (odds ratio 0.25; confidence interval 0.13–0.48),[37] and this finding supports long-term treatment in patients with extensive colitis.

Treatment of active disease

Higher doses of 5-ASA (4 g/day) have a role for inducing remission in both mild UC and CD. The emphasis should be on the "mild" condition. In Crohn's ileitis, Pentasa at 4 g daily for 16 weeks induced remission in 43% of 75 patients, compared with 23% of 80 subjects who received placebo; the number needed to treat (NNT) to achieve one remission was 4.[38] In UC, greater clinical improvement, but not necessarily disease remission, is associated with doses greater or equal to 3 g/day (70% of patients improved, but only 30–50% of entered remission within 8 weeks of 5-ASA therapy). Clinical improvement characteristically occurs at twice the remission rate. This is demonstrated by the findings from the most recent meta-analysis of oral 5-ASA compounds for active disease.[34] Of 19 trials involving 2032 patients, nine were placebo-controlled and 10 compared mesalazine with sulfasalazine.[34] Based on an intention-to-treat principle, the outcome of interest in the treatment of active disease was the failure to induce remission; the difference between two treatments was indicated by the pooled Peto odds ratio (a pooled odds ratio < 1.0 indicated that one treatment was more effective than another; the lower the value, the more significant difference between treatments). The findings from this meta-analysis showed that mesalazine was more than twice as effective as placebo (odds ration 0.39; confidence interval 0.29–0.52), but was not significantly better than sulfasalazine (odds ration 0.87; confidence interval 0.63–1.20).

Adverse effects

Side effects of sulfasalazine occur in 10–30% of treated patients, depending on the dose. The side-effects of new 5-ASAs do not differ significantly between drugs (*see Appendix 1* and Loftus EV, Kane SV, Bjorkman D. Systematic review: short term adverse effects of 5-aminosalicyclic acid agents in ulcerative colitis. *Aliment Pharmacol Ther* 2004:**19**:179-89). Intolerance to mesalazine occurs in up to 15% of treated patients. Acute intolerance is rarer (3%) and may be difficult to distinguish from a flare of colitis since it includes bloody diarrhoea. Its recurrence on re-challenge provides the clue if the patient has not already suspected it; clinicians, however, should be aware that 5-ASA can occasionally exacerbate the colitis.

Corticosteroids

Choice and mechanism

Corticosteroids form the cornerstone for inducing remission in both UC and CD. They have no role in maintenance therapy for either disease. Their mechanism of action is to inhibit several inflammatory pathways – suppression of mRNA that transcribes interleukins; induction of IκB that stabilizes the NFκB complex, which upregulates the inflammatory response; suppression of arachidonic acid metabolism; and stimulation of apoptosis of lymphocytes within the lamina propria of the gut.[39]

Efficacy for active Crohn's disease

Two major multicentre trials established corticosteroids as the most effective therapy for inducing remission in CD. In the National Co-operative Crohn's Disease Study (162 randomized patients), 60% remission was achieved with prednisone (0.5–0.75 mg/kg/day – the higher dose for more severe disease and tapering over 17 weeks), compared with 30% remission in patients on placebo (NNT = 3).[40] In a comparable study, the European Cooperative Crohn's Disease Study (105 randomized patients), 83% remission was achieved with prednisone (1 mg/kg/day), compared with 38% remission in the placebo group (NNT = 2), over 18 weeks.[41] The high-placebo response rate should be noted because disease activity in CD, and UC, fluctuates spontaneously. Although no formal dose-response trial has been performed, 92% remission was achieved within 7 weeks in 142 patients with moderately active CD treated with prednisone (1 mg/kg/day, without tapering).[42]

Efficacy for active ulcerative colitis

The same observation applies to induction of remission in UC. Although trials are all over 30 years old, the results are consistent. Oral prednisolone (starting at 40 mg/day) induced remission in 77% of 118 patients with mild-to-moderate disease within 2 weeks, compared to 48% treated with 8 g/day sulfasalazine.[43] A combination of oral and rectal steroids is better than treatment with either drug alone.[44] Adverse events are significantly more frequent at a dose of 60 mg/day compared with 40mg/day, without added benefit.[45] Thus, 40 mg/day appears optimal for out-patient management of acute UC. Too rapid a reduction in the treatment dose can be associated with early relapse, and doses of prednisolone lower than of equal to15 mg/day are ineffective for active disease.[45]

Treatment decision with steroids

The efficacy of steroids has to be balanced against their side effects (*see* later in this section), but it is helpful to discuss risks *versus* benefits with patients who are often naturally disposed against steroids. It is important that treatment decisions of active disease are made in conjunction with the patient, with a strategy for complete withdrawal of steroids. A patient who suffers miserable symptoms from IBD often appreciates decisive treatment with steroids.

Steroid regimen[46]

Regimens of steroid therapy vary between centres, but it is helpful to use a standard weaning strategy because this approach allow the identification of patients who relapse rapidly or do not respond to treatment. These patients will then need adjunctive therapy either with AZA or as an in-patient procedure. The strategy used at the John Radcliffe Hospital, Oxford, is shown in Table 7.

Adverse effects

Potential side effects of steroids are a real concern; however, 50% of patients do not experience any adverse event. Besides some inconveniences from a cosmetic viewpoint (e.g. acne, moon face or oedema), the most commonly reported adverse effects are sleep and mood disturbance. Nevertheless, it is those adverse events associated with prolonged use (>12 weeks usually, but sometimes less) that are best avoided by withdrawing steroids. These include osteoporosis, osteonecrosis of the femoral head, myopathy and fragile skin. Although not technically a side effect, a consequence of long-term treatment with steroids (> 3 months) is to cause withdrawal syndrome of myalgia, malaise and arthralgia, which is not dissimilar to a recrudescence of CD. Withdrawal is best achieved by early introduction of AZA, nutritional therapy or timely surgery (*see Surgical therapy in inflammatory bowel diseases*). The fact that steroids have no place in preventing relapse of UC or CD should be emphasized, and if patient cannot be weaned off steroids then

Table 7. Treatment of active ulcerative colitis after topical mesalazine (1 g/day) for up to 2 weeks

Drug	Mild	Moderate	Severe
Prednisolone	20 mg/day for 1 month	40 mg/day for 1 week	Admit for iv steroids
	15 mg/day for 1 week	30 mg/day for 1 week	Telephone gastroenterologist
	10 mg/day for 1 week	Then as for mild attacks	
	5 mg/day for 1 week		
Aminosalicylates	Oral mesalazine 2–4 g/day, balsalazide 6.75 g/day or olsalazine 1.5–3 g/day	As for mild attacks	None until oral therapy restarted
	Review after 2 weeks; if active disease remains, then treat with oral prednisolone and review after 2–4 weeks	As for mild attacks	
Enemas	Mesalazine 1 g/day while bleeding		

specialist reassessment, at a referral centre if necessary, is appropriate.

Topical therapy

General

Topical therapy makes sense in distal colitis or proctitis. Enemas or suppositories deliver high drug concentrations to the site of inflammation and minimize systemic absorption.

Site of action

Isotope scintigraphy shows that suppositories coat the distal 20 cm of rectum, foam enemas reach the descending colon and 100-ml liquid enemas can reach the splenic flexure.

Proximal distribution is aided by reflex rectal contraction, but this contraction can also overcome anal sphincter pressure and this means that some patients cannot retain enemas.

Tolerability and preference
Patients tolerate solid suppositories better than foam, and foam better than liquid. Applicators and manual dexterity also affect individual choice. Furthermore, less than 10% of liquid enemas and less than 40% of foam enemas remain in the rectum at 4 hours, so suppositories are preferable if disease is limited to the rectum.

Choice of topical therapy
The choice of topical therapy should be made by taking into consideration the disease distribution (proctitis, distal or more extensive), and treatment activity (sole therapy or as an adjunct to systemic therapy) and efficacy (topical mesalazine is more effective than steroid). It is logical to combine suppositories with enemas, as there is limited evidence that combining topical steroid and mesalazine is effective for refractory left-sided or distal colitis.[47]

Topical steroids
Four types are marketed in the UK: hydrocortisone (Colifoam®); prednisolone metasulphobenzoate (Predenema® 100-ml enema or Predfoam®); prednisolone phosphate (Predsol® 100 ml or suppository) and budesonide (100-ml enema).

Systemic effect
Absorption, and therefore the degree of adrenal suppression, depends on retention time, degree of inflammation and drug type. Prednisolone metasulpho-benzoate and budesonide cause less adrenal suppression, but this is of biochemical, rather than clinical, relevance.[47]

Efficacy and choice
All topical steroids are modestly effective for active distal UC. In a study of 233 patients, remission rates at 8 weeks

with budesonide enemas were 19% (2 mg) and 27% (8 mg), compared with 4% in placebo-treated patients.[48] In a meta-analysis of rectal corticosteroids in conjunction with oral 5-ASA, pooled remission rates by symptomatic, endoscopic and histological criteria were 45%, 34% and 29%, respectively, up to 8 weeks.[49] Placebo remission rates were 9% and 17% by symptomatic and endoscopic criteria. The cost of budesonide enemas (approx. £120/month, compared with £15 for Colifoam® or Predsol®) is difficult to justify given these modest results.

Role

All topical steroids should be used as an adjunct to oral therapy in active distal colitis, usually twice-daily while visible bleeding is present, then once at night for 2 weeks. They are less effective than topical 5-ASA, but some patients find them easier to tolerate.

Topical 5-aminosalicylates

Three types are marketed in the UK: Pentasa® (100-ml enema or 1-g suppository); Asacol® (foam or 500-mg suppository) and Salofalk® (2-g 60-ml enema, 1-g foam or 500-mg suppository).

Efficacy and choice

Dose-ranging studies confirm that 1 g is as effective as 2 or 4 g, with remission rates after 30 days of 63%, 67% and 72%, respectively, in 113 patients.[50] Furthermore, a single high-dose suppository (Pentasa 1 g) was more rapidly effective than two 500-mg suppositories (Claversal, similar to Salofalk) twice-daily for inducing remission in 51 patients with active proctitis.[51] Within 2 weeks of treatment, clinical (and endoscopic) remission occured in 64% (52%) of patients on Pentasa, compared with 28% (24%) of patients on Claversal suppositories ($P < 0.01$). Consequently, 1-g suppositories are favoured over 500-mg suppositories.

Comparison with topical steroids

There is clear evidence that topical mesalazine is more effective than topical steroids. The pooled odds ratio comparing the two treatments in seven trials showed rectal 5-ASA to be superior for disease remission, whether it be for symptoms (odds ratio 2.42; confidence interval 1.72–3.41), endoscopy (odds ratio 1.89; confidence interval 1.29–2.76) or histology (odds ratio 2.03; confidence intervals 1.28–3.20).[49]

Role

Topical 5-ASA should therefore be the treatment of first choice in active distal UC. Although there is no evidence from controlled trials in Crohn's proctitis, suppositories for local active CD are worth trying. Topical 5-ASA is also useful for maintaining remission, but is generally less acceptable than oral therapy. Mesalazine 1-g suppositories (Pentasa) three times a week maintained remission in 52% of treated patients over 1 year, compared with 38% in the placebo group ($P = 0.018$).[52] Increasing the dose to 1g/day induced remission in 61% of those who relapsed within 30 days, compared with 8% of those given placebo. Consequently, when oral salicylates alone fail, Pentasa® 1-g suppositories three times weekly are appropriate for maintaining remission in refractory proctitis.

Antibiotics in Crohn's disease

Antibiotics are frequently used in CD, especially if fistulae or other infective complications occur, but rarely as monotherapy.

Evidence

In the largest study to date, metronidazole was no more effective than placebo at inducing remission, although there was a significant ($P = 0.002$) improvement in disease activity compared with placebo.[53] Ciprofloxacin has been reported to be as effective as mesalazine,[54] but one suspects that the response of apparently active disease to antibiotics is often seen because diarrhoea is due to intestinal bacterial overgrowth.

Antimycobacterial therapy

Three trials on the use of antimycobacterial chemotherapy (using different combinations of ethambutol, rifampicin, isoniazid, sulphadoxine and pyrimethamine) to induce remission have failed to show benefit over placebo. The findings of a large trial of quadruple therapy are expected in 2004. However, two of six trials that used steroids to induce remission showed that antimycobacterial therapy helped prevent relapse.[55]

Current indications

Metronidazole, or ciprofloxacin, for CD is therefore reserved for suspected bacterial overgrowth (characterized by explosive diarrhoea with little abdominal pain) or perianal disease, and only for primary treatment of mild ileitis if a patient is intolerant to more effective therapy.

Immunomodulatory therapy

Azathioprine and mercaptopurine

Thiopurines (AZA and MP) are effective for both inducing remission of active disease and maintaining remission in both CD and UC.

Evidence

A Cochrane review of the efficacy of AZA and MP in inducing remission of active CD demonstrated a benefit for thiopurine therapy compared with placebo (odds ratio 2.36; 95% confidence interval 1.57–3.53).[56] This equates to an NNT of 5 and a number needed to harm (NNH) of 14. Their efficacy in maintaining remission is confirmed in another Cochrane review (odds ratio 2.16; confidence interval 1.35–3.47; NNT = 7).[57]

Azathioprine or mercaptopurine?

For historical reasons AZA has been the choice of clinicians in Europe, while MP is exclusively used in parts of America. There are no direct comparisons of the efficacy of AZA and MP in IBD. Nevertheless, patients who are intolerant of AZA can frequently tolerate MP.[58]

Indication for thiopurines

The main role for AZA or MP as steroid sparing agents in CD has been demonstrated (odds ratio 5.22; confidence interval 1.06–25.68; NNT = 3),[57] and should be considered at an early stage in those patients whose symptoms recur as the dose of prednisolone is tapered, or recur soon after prednisolone is stopped. For arbitrary but practical purposes, this approach also applies to UC and means that:

- patients who require two or more courses of corticosteroids within a calendar year
- patients whose disease relapses as the dose of steroid is reduced below 15 mg
- relapse within 6 weeks of stopping steroid
- postoperative prophylaxis of complex (fistulating or extensive) CD.

Duration of therapy

The published evidence suggests that thiopurines are effective as maintenance therapy for CD for up to 4 years. In a prospective trial, 83 patients with CD who had been in remission for 3.5 years on AZA were randomized to continue AZA or placebo and followed up for 18 months. The relapse rates were 21% and 8% in the placebo and AZA groups, respectively ($P = 0.0195$). Practical advice for patients with either CD or UC who are started on AZA is to continue treatment for 3–4 years and then stop, except in those with evidence of continuing disease activity. For the 20% of patients who relapse, AZA should be restarted and continued.

Dosing

Tailoring or optimization of thiopurine therapy can occur prior to, or during, treatment. Clinicians should aim for a maintenance dose of AZA of 2–2.5 mg/kg/day and MP of 1–1.5 mg/kg/day in both UC and CD. The "maximum" dose differs between individuals and effectively means the level at which leucopenia develops. Leucopenia is a myelotoxic side effect of thiopurines, and the metabolic phenotype of the individual can be defined by measuring thiopurine methyl transferase (TPMT) activity or the TPMT genotype.

Is measurement of TPMT necessary?

Individuals who are TPMT-deficient are at increased risk of myelotoxicity.[59] The problem is that it does not necessarily apply in IBD. In one study, the majority (77%) of 41 patients with AZA-induced bone marrow suppression did not carry a TPMT mutation,[60] and evidence that TPMT activity predicts other side effects or outcome is slender.[61] TPMT measurement cannot yet be recommended as a pre-requisite to therapy, since decades of experience has shown clinical AZA to be safe in UC or CD.[62]

Monitoring thiopurine therapy

The manufacturers of AZA recommend weekly FBCs for the first 8 weeks of therapy, followed by FBCs at least every 3 months thereafter. There is no evidence that this is effective. The authors' practice is to perform an FBC every 2–4 weeks for 2 months and then every 8–12 weeks. The rationale for this approach is that about half the patients who develop myelotoxicity will develop it within 2 months and nearly two-thirds within 4 months.[60] Just as important is the advice to patients to report promptly should a sore throat, or any other sign of infection, occur. (*See* Table 8 for a summary of monitoring recommendations.)

Side effects

Profound leucopenia can develop suddenly and unpredictably, in-between blood tests, although patients (and their GPs) should be reassured that it is rare (around 3% of patients overall). Hepatotoxicity and pancreatitis are also uncommon (< 5%). Much more common are flu-like symptoms (myalgia, headache or diarrhoea) that characteristically occur 2–3 weeks after starting AZA but cease rapidly when the drug is withdrawn. Although it is the best agent for maintaining remission, clinical findings showed that 28% of 622 patients experienced side effects.[62] Fortunately, when the drug is tolerated for 3 weeks, long-term benefit can be expected.

Thiopurines in pregnancy

There are two other concerns with thiopurines. One is safety in pregnancy and the other is whether it increases the risk of lymphoma. For women with IBD who are maintained on a thiopurine and are considering conception, the authors' advice is usually to continue therapy through pregnancy. This advice is based on a study of 155 men and women with IBD who were parents of 347 pregnancies while taking MP.[63] The authors of this study found no difference in miscarriage, congenital abnormality or infection rate in the thiopurine group compared with the control group.[63]

Thiopurines and lymphoma

Large audits from John Radcliffe Hospital, Oxford (622 patients)[62] and St Mark's Hospital, London (755 patients)[64] have shown no increased risk of lymphoma or other cancers in IBD patients treated with AZA. A primary care prescribing database study of nearly 1,500 IBD patients who received at least one prescription of AZA/6-MP also showed no overall risk (relative risk 1.6; 95% confidence interval 0.1–8.8) of lymphoma, but little is known about the duration or dose of therapy of this cohort.[65] A decision analysis suggests that the benefits of AZA outweighs the small risk of lymphoma in IBD.[66]

Methotrexate

MTX is an effective treatment for inducing remission or preventing relapse in CD. At present, the role of MTX is in the treatment of active or relapsing CD in patients who are refractory, or intolerant to, AZA or MP.

Evidence in Crohn's disease

In a controlled study, Feagan *et al*. randomized 141 steroid-dependent patients to either 25 mg/week of intramuscular MTX or placebo for 16 weeks, with a concomitant daily dose of prednisolone (20 mg at initiation) that was reduced over a 3-month period.[67] Significantly more patients in the MTX-treated group were able to withdraw steroids and enter remission compared with placebo (39% *vs* 19%; $P = 0.025$); no serious toxicity was reported. In a subsequent study, a MTX, at a smaller dose, was shown to be effective at preventing relapse after remission of CD had been induced by this drug at a higher dose. After entering remission induced by treatment with intramuscular MTX at 25 mg/week, 76 patients were randomized to either MTX (15 mg/week) or placebo for 9 months.[68] At week 40, MTX was more efficient than placebo in maintaining remission (65% *vs* 39%; $P = 0.04$) and reducing the need for steroids caused by relapse (28% *vs* 58%; $P = 0.01$).

Evidence in ulcerative colitis

In contrast to its role in CD, few trials have addressed the role of MTX in either the induction or the maintenance of remission in UC. The initial report by Kozarek in 1989 showed that MTX induced remission in five of seven patients with UC.[69] Oren *et al*. conducted the study in 67 patients with UC who were randomized to oral MTX (12.5 mg/week) or placebo for 9 months, and found no difference in the induction or maintenance of remission.[70] However, a retrospective review of clinical notes taken from 22 patients with UC and 48 patients with CD indicated that the remission rates, and maintenance of remission, were similar between these two groups treated with similar doses of MTX (median 22.5mg/week).[71]

Dose and delivery[70]
The dose and route of administration of MTX may be both important factors in the induction of remission.[72] Unlike rheumatoid arthritis, doses smaller than 15 mg/day are ineffective, and 25 mg/day is the standard dose for CD. For practical reasons relating to the reconstitution of parenteral cytotoxic drugs, oral dosing is far more convenient than subcutaneous administration, which is restricted to patients with small intestinal CD who do not absorb oral MTX.

Duration of therapy
The duration of therapy is debated. The 3-year remission rate for MTX obtained by Fraser et al. was 51%[71] and compares well with that of AZA (69%) obtained by the same authors.[62]

Side effects
Early toxicity from MTX is primarily gastrointestinal (nausea, vomiting, diarrhoea and stomatitis), and this can be limited by co-prescription of folic acid 5 mg 2 or 3 days apart from MTX. A convenient way to remember this is: "**M**TX on a **M**onday and **F**olic acid on a **F**riday". Treatment is discontinued in 10–18% of patients because of side effects.[71] The principal concerns are hepatotoxicity and pneumonitis. A study of liver biopsies in IBD patients on MTX showed mostly only mild histologic abnormalities, despite cumulative doses of up to 5410 mg.[73] Surveillance liver biopsy is not warranted, but if the aspartate aminotransferase level doubles then it is sensible to withhold MTX until this level returns to normal before a re-challenge. The prevalence of pneumonitis has been estimated to be two to three cases per 100 patient-years of exposure, but some case series have not reported any.[74] (*See* Table 8 for a summary of monitoring recommendations.)

Ciclosporin

CsA is a fungal metabolite and powerful immunomodulator that inhibits calcineurin, a phosphatase involved in the function of T helper cells and recruitment of cytotoxic T cell populations.[75]

Therapeutic value

Intravenous CsA is rapidly effective as a salvage therapy for patients with refractory colitis who would otherwise face colectomy, but its use is controversial because of toxicity and long-term failure rate. Toxicity can be reduced by using lower intravenous CsA doses (2 mg/kg/day),[76] oral micro-emulsion CsA[77] or CsA monotherapy without corticosteroids.[78] The drug should not be continued for more than 3 to 6 months, and its main role is as a bridge to AZA or MP.[79] A meta-analysis of four randomized controlled trials has shown that CsA has no therapeutic value in CD.[80]

Evidence

CsA is normally initiated in hospital for severe UC refractory to intravenous steroids.[81] In the single placebo-controlled trial, 20 patients were randomized to intravenous CsA (4 mg/kg/day) or placebo in addition to continued glucocorticoids for up to 14 days.[82] Nine out of 11 patients treated with CsA improved after 7 days compared with none out of 9 patients given placebo, of whom seven subsequently responded to treatment when given open-label CsA. Uncontrolled trials confirmed the promising initial response rates of 82% at day 7, and 69% at 6 months.[82;83] Successful treatment with CsA avoids the immediate necessity of a surgical procedure, but the relapse and colectomy rates may subsequently be high. At the John Radcliffe Hospital, Oxford, 58% of 76 patients with severe, refractory UC treated with CsA came to colectomy after 7 years (Campbell *et al.*, 2004, unpublished data).

Side effects

To reduce this high relapse rate, oral AZA is usually introduced after remission has been achieved with CsA.[84;85] Serious concerns remain about side effects including opportunistic infection such as *Pneumocystis carinii* pneumonia. Minor side effects occur in 31–51% of treated patients, including tremor, paraesthesiae, malaise, headache, abnormal liver function, gingival hyperplasia and hirsutism. Major complications have been reported in 0–17% of treated patients, including renal impairment, infections and neurotoxicity.[81]

Monitoring
Monitoring after discharge from hospital best includes the measurement of blood pressure, creatinine level and blood CsA concentration (target: 100–200 ng/ml) every 2–4 weeks (Table 8).

Nutritional therapy

For CD, nutrition should be considered as an integral component of the management of all patients. Malnutrition is common and multifactorial in origin (Table 9). Nutritional status (including body mass index) is best assessed at diagnosis, and periodically thereafter. As a minimum, patients should be weighed on out-patient attendance or in primary care. In children and adolescents, regular monitoring with height and weight centile charts is mandatory. Nutritional therapy can be considered as disease-modifying, or adjunctive, therapy.[86]

Disease-modifying therapy
Efficacy
Enteral nutrition is undoubtedly less effective than steroids as primary treatment for CD (Figure 8), but the argument is becoming more about safety than efficacy. Three published meta-analyses and a Cochrane Database Systematic review[87] have confirmed that steroids are more effective than enteral nutrition for inducing remission. Based on the principle of intention-to-treat, the NNT to induce remission with steroids, instead of enteral nutrition, is 4. This can be compared with an NNT to induce remission with steroids, instead of placebo, of 3. So far, no placebo-controlled trial has been conducted with enteral nutrition.

Table 8. Summary of monitoring recommendations for immunomodulator therapy[*†‡]

Drug	Full blood count	Liver function tests	Action if deranged
Azathioprine	0, 2, 4 and 8 weeks, then every 8–12 weeks	0 and 4 weeks, then every 6 months	*WBC 3.5–4.0:* recheck at 2 weeks *WBC 3.0–3.5:* halve dose; recheck at 1 week; restart at half dose when WBC > 3.5 *WBC 2.0–3.0:* stop drug; recheck weekly; do not restart until specialist advice *WBC < 2.0:* stop drug and telephone gastroenterologist
Mercaptopurine	As for azathioprine	As for azathioprine	As for azathioprine Note that macrocytosis is usual (as for azathioprine)
Methotrexate	0 and 4 weeks, then monthly	0 and 4 weeks then monthly	If ALT < 2-fold elevated, recheck monthly If ALT > 2-fold elevated, stop drug and contact gastroenterologist
Ciclosporin	**Blood pressure**	**Creatinine**	**Ciclosporin concentration**
	4-weekly	4-weekly	1, 2, 4 and 8 weeks; aim 100–200 ng/ml

*Patients on immunomodulators for inflammatory bowel diseases are less susceptible to myelotoxicity than patients with rheumatoid arthritis.
†Monitoring recommendations have no evidence base, and leucopenia (for instance) can occur within days of a previously normal count.
‡Recommendations above are a pragmatic guide, as practised in Oxford.
Patients should be advised to seek prompt medical help if a sore throat, fever or other systemic symptoms develop.
WBC = white blood cells; ALT = alanine transaminase

Table 9. Frequency of different nutritional deficiencies in inflammatory bowel disease*†

Type of deficiency	Frequency of deficiency (%)
Growth retardation	20–40
Final height < 5th percentile	7–30
Weight loss (active phase)	75
Loss of muscle mass/fat mass	60
Osteopenia	45
Iron deficiency/anemia	70
Vitamin D deficiency	~ 50
Deficiency in K, Ca, PO₄, MG	Described
Deficiency in fat-soluble vitamins/vitamin B₁₂	Described
Folic acid deficiency	Described

*Data taken from published literature.
†Reproduced with permission from Lochs H. Nutrition in inflammatory bowel disease. In: *Kirsner's inflammatory bowel diseases*, edited by R Balfour Sartor and WJ Sandborn. Edinburgh: Saunders. 2004.

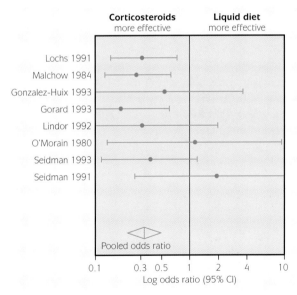

Figure 8. Efficacy of corticosteroids compared with that of liquid diets in Crohn's disease (data taken from published literature). Reproduced with permission from Gassull MA, Stange EF. Nutrition and diet in inflammatory bowel disease. In: Inflammatory bowel diseases, edited by J Satsangi and LR Sutherland. Edinburgh: Churchill Livingstone. 2003.

Selection of patients

Nutritional therapy is appropriate for growth failure in children or adolescents with active small bowel disease. In adolescents with CD, enteral nutrition allows normal growth and sexual development, and may also maintain remission.[88;89] The decision on its use is made after detailed discussion with the patient. Enteral nutrition may be preferred to steroids, immunomodulators or surgery in any patient with active disease, in patients who are unresponsive to mesalazine or those in whom corticosteroids are contraindicated. Careful selection of highly motivated patients, and strong support from (highly) motivated dieticians and doctors, for both treatment and weaning period improves outcome. The recommended uses of nutritional therapy are summarized in Table 10.

Choice of feed

The choice of liquid feed (polymeric, oligopeptide or elemental) matters less than compliance. Feed (un)palatability, a slower response than steroids, an inability to stay on a solid-free diet for 6 or more weeks, social inconvenience and transient food-related adverse reactions, all contribute to poor compliance. Up to 40% of patients find it impossible to comply with their diet.

Adjunctive therapy

Selection

Nutritional support is appropriate as adjunctive therapy for any malnourished patient or patients who have difficulty to maintain a normal nutritional status.[90] It is appropriate for

---

Table 10. Recommended uses of nutritional therapy

Nutritional therapy is appropriate for:

- Growth retardation in children or adolescents with active small bowel disease
- Highly motivated patients with active small bowel disease (after detailed discussion and careful selection)
- Patients in whom corticosteroids are contraindicated
- Adjuvant therapy with medication, especially prior to surgery.

patients with partial intestinal obstruction awaiting surgery, or those with severely symptomatic perianal disease or postoperative complications.

General dietary advice for patients with Crohn's disease
Most patients can eat anything. Patients should avoid foods that upset them and try to adopt a balanced diet. Many patients find that avoiding vegetables and other foods high in fibre relieve abdominal pain during an acute episode, especially if there is small intestinal disease. Patients usually find it helpful to see a dietician at diagnosis, who can ensure that calcium or iron intake is not inappropriately restricted. Wrong advice to avoid dairy products is commonplace and this limits calcium intake.

Nutrition and ulcerative colitis
There is little evidence to implicate dietary components in the aetiology or pathogenesis of UC. However, patients are prone to malnutrition and its detrimental effects. In contrast to CD, there is no evidence that artificial nutritional support alters the inflammatory response in UC.

Infliximab

Tumour necrosis factor plays a pivotal role in mucosal inflammation. IFX is a chimeric anti-tumour necrosis factor (anti-TNF) monoclonal antibody with potent anti-inflammatory effects, probably based on apoptosis of inflammatory cells. Numerous controlled trials have demonstrated its efficacy in both active and fistulating CD.

Evidence in inflammatory Crohn's disease
The findings from a multicentre, double-blind study in 108 patients with moderate-to-severe CD refractory to 5-ASA, corticosteroids and/or immunomodulators showed an 81% response rate after 4 weeks of treatment with 5 mg/kg IFX, compared with 17% in the placebo group.[91] The duration of response varied considerably, but 48 % of the patients who were treated with IFX still showed a response at week 12.

The ACCENT-1 study,[92] the definitive re-treatment trial, was conducted to evaluate maintenance of remission in 335, out of an initial 573, patients with active CD who had responded to a single infusion of IFX at 5 mg/kg. This study had a complex protocol, and patients were treated with either placebo or IFX (5 or 10 mg/kg) every 8 weeks until week 46. At week 30, 21% of the patients on placebo were in remission compared with 39 % and 45% of patients treated with 5 mg/kg IFX ($P = 0.003$) and 10 mg/kg IFX ($P = 0.0002$), respectively. These findings indicate that the initial response to IFX infusion could be maintained over a longer period if treatment was repeated every 8 weeks, although more than half of the treated patients relapsed in spite of maintenance IFX infusions.

Evidence in fistulating Crohn's disease

Perianal or other types of fistulas are observed at some time during the disease history in 20–45 % of patients. The classic medical treatment based on antibiotics and immunosuppressive drugs has been disappointing, and a multidisciplinary approach with surgical input is mandatory. IFX is the first agent to show a therapeutic effect in a controlled trial. Ninety-four patients with draining abdominal or perianal fistulas of at least 3 months in duration were treated. Of the treated patients, 68% in the 5 mg/kg group and 56% in the 10 mg/kg group experienced a reduction in the number of draining fistulas at two or more consecutive visits, compared with 26% for placebo ($P = 0.002$ and 0.02, respectively). The duration of this effect was, however, limited in most cases to only 3 or 4 months.[93] To investigate the long-term effect of IFX on fistulating CD, a large maintenance trial (ACCENT-II) was performed.[94] Three hundred and six patients with actively draining enterocutaneous fistulae were treated with three induction infusions of IFX (5 mg/kg) at week 0, 2 and 6. One hundred and ninety-five out of 306 patients (69%) showed a response to treatment, and were subsequently randomized to maintenance infusion (5 mg/kg IFX) or placebo every 8 weeks. Those who lost their response to treatment were either switched from placebo to active treatment (5 mg/kg IFX), or had their re-treatment dose increased from 5 to 10 mg/kg IFX, every 8 weeks. At the end of the 12-month trial, 46% of patients on active re-treatment showed a fistula response compared with 23% for placebo ($P = 0.001$), and complete closure of fistulae was observed in 36 % of patients on active treatment compared with 19 % for placebo ($P = 0.009$).

Selection
National guidelines govern the use of IFX. In the UK, this use is limited to patients with severe active CD (HBI > 8; CDAI > 300) who are refractory, or intolerant, to steroids and immunomodulators and for whom surgery is inappropriate. Criteria are less exacting in the US and some European countries, despite the fact that aminosalicylates or antibiotics are acceptable indications for active disease. Retreatment is usually necessary after a variable interval (most commonly 8–16 weeks). Unless there is intolerance, all patients should receive an immunomodulator (AZA, MP or MTX), as this probably extends the treatment interval and reduces the development of antibodies to IFX, which, in turn, reduce the efficacy and increase the side effects. In the UK, "maintenance" IFX is not yet approved by NICE and re-treatment is only given for recurrent active disease.

Side effects
After initial concerns, it is now clear that IFX treatment is relatively safe if used for appropriate indications. Infusion reactions during, or shortly after, infusion are rare and respond to slowing the infusion rate or treatment with antihistamines, paracetamol and, sometimes, corticosteroids. The majority of symptoms are "allergic", including rash, hypotension, shortness of breath and low-grade fever. Anaphylactic reactions have been reported. A delayed reaction of joint pain and stiffness, fever, myalgia and malaise may occur if there has been an interval longer than 1 year following a previous infusion. All patients recovered with antihistamines and corticosteroids.

Safety

Infection is the main concern. Active sepsis (e.g. abscess) is an absolute contraindication since this increases the risk of overwhelming septicaemia. Reactivation, or development, of tuberculosis is also a major concern.[94;95] The risk depends partly on the geographical prevalence of tuberculosis. Screening for earlier exposure by chest x-ray seems mandatory but insensitive. Skin testing cannot be relied upon because it is often negative owing to anergy or immunosuppression in patients with active CD. IFX can also exacerbate existing cardiac failure. The major theoretical worry is that of lymphoproliferative disorders since endogenous TNF is likely to have a role in tumour suppression. Five lymphoproliferative disorders were reported in the initial controlled clinical trials of IFX for rheumatoid arthritis and CD. However, post-marketing surveillance has not corroborated this risk after more than 500,000 infusions have been performed in the US and Europe, although with short follow-up.

Practical issues

Intravenous infusions of IFX are given over 2 hr, usually as an out-patient procedure. Pulse rate and blood pressure 30 min to 2hr after the infusion are customary. Patients should understand that IFX is a novel therapy, which is usually effective for only 12–16 weeks and is primarily designed to induce remission while immunomodulators alter the pattern of disease. If patients fail to respond or lose their response, referral to a specialist centre is appropriate for nutritional therapy, surgery or consideration of other new biological therapy.

Clinical problem: treating acute relapses of ulcerative colitis or Crohn's disease

The principles for both UC and CD are to confirm disease activity, assess the severity and consider the location.

For all patients

History should be taken (stool frequency, onset of symptoms within a day is more likely to be due to infection than active disease, lack of bleeding virtually excludes active UC), the patient should be examined for pulse rate, abdominal tenderness and temperature, FBC and CRP should be checked. For symptoms of short duration (< 3 weeks), stool culture should be obtained and *Cl. difficile* toxin assay requested. For patients with UC, a proctoscopy should be performed. The principal steps to exclude or confirm active disease are summarized in Table 11.

Table 11. Principal steps to exclude/ confirm active disease

For all patients:

History
- Stool frequency
- Symptoms
  - Onset within 1 day suggests infection
- Bleeding
  - No blood in stool suggests infection

Examination
- Pulse rate
- Abdominal tenderness
- Temperature

Blood tests/laboratory tests
- Full blood count
- C-reactive protein level
- *C. difficile* toxin assay from stool culture
  (if symptom duration < 3 weeks)

Proctoscopy
- Proctoscopy **and biopsy** if ulcerative colitis is **suspected**

Mild-to-moderate distal ulcerative colitis

It is characterized by bloody stool frequency less than six times a day without a tachycardia or temperature. Topical mesalazine 1g/day (suppositories for proctitis, foam enemas for distal disease) should be started, combined with oral mesalazine 2–4 g/day, olsalazine 1.5–3 g/day or balsalazide 6.75 g/day, followed by a review of the patient's condition in 2 weeks. Patients who still have active disease after a fortnight should be treated with oral prednisolone (Table 7). Review in 2–4 weeks. After remission has been achieved, the role and importance of maintenance therapy using 5-ASA should be discussed with the patient.

Mild-to-moderate extensive ulcerative colitis

Prednisolone should be started when UC is first diagnosed. The risk of under-treatment and toxic dilatation is higher than that of distal UC.

Severe ulcerative colitis

It is characterized by bloody stool frequency more than six times a day, with one or more of the following findings: a tachycardia (pulse rate > 90 bpm); temperature (> 37.5°C); anaemia (haemoglobin [Hb] < 10.5 g/dl; ESR > 30mm/hr or CRP > 50 mg/l (*see* Table 3 of section *Introduction and background*). Telephone the gastro-enterologist in charge to arrange admission for intensive treatment as 30% of patients with severe UC will undergo colectomy on that admission.[96] Remember that patients with severe UC may look deceptively well.

Mild-to-moderate ileal or ileocolic Crohn's disease

The patient is ambulatory, and eating and drinking are normal, without fever, tachycardia, dehydration or signs of obstruction, and weight loss is less than 10%. Treatment and previous response to treatment should be discussed with the patient. Corticosteroids remain the mainstay, starting with prednisolone at 40 mg/day for 1 week, then 30 mg/day for 1 week and followed by 20 mg/day for 1 month before decreasing the dose by 5 mg/day each week). 5-ASAs (e.g. Pentasa 4 g/day) are an alternative for mild symptoms that are not interfering with daily activity. Budesonide (starting at 9 mg/d for 6 weeks, then 6 mg/day for 4 weeks) is an alternative for ileo-ascending colonic disease if patients are intolerant to steroids, but works less well than prednisolone. Strategies to prevent relapse, when reviewed, should be discussed with the patient, especially the importance of stopping smoking.

Mild-to-moderate colonic Crohn's disease
High-dose 5-ASA is ineffective and prednisolone should be started when first seen. Care should be taken to check the date of the last relapse and steroid treatment, because AZA may need to be started as well (*see Medical therapy – Therapeutic strategy*).

Severe ileal or colonic Crohn's disease
Severe ileal or colonic CD is suspected when treatment for mild-to-moderate disease is ineffective, or one or more of the following symptoms is observed: vomiting, dehydration, tachycardia, fever, tender mass, or weight loss > 10%. Telephone the gastroenterologist in charge to discuss admission. If there is any possibility of obstruction, prompt referral to hospital should be made.

Surgical therapy in inflammatory bowel diseases

Ulcerative colitis

Colectomy is the only cure for UC, although it does not affect some of the extra-intestinal manifestations such as hepatobiliary disease or AS.

Indications

Colectomy is usually indicated for extensive disease, but is occasionally needed for distal colitis. Indications for surgery in UC are:

- Failure of medical treatment (chronic, continuous symptoms or side effects)
- Severe colitis not responding to intensive treatment
- Complications (dysplasia or cancer, colonic dilatation, perforation or massive haemorrhage).

Operation

Colectomy with a temporary ileostomy and later ileo-anal pouch construction is now the operation of choice but proctocolectomy, followed by permanent ileostomy, retains a definite place. The patient should see a stomatherapist and may want to talk to an ileostomist of the same gender, and similar age, before surgery.

Proctocolectomy and ileostomy

The diseased colon is removed in its entirety. This procedure provides a definitive cure but with the encumbrance of a long-term ileostomy. It is usually performed in two stages (subtotal colectomy and, later, proctectomy after an interval of some months), unless the patient is in a good nutritional state, and the decision about a permanent ileostomy is unequivocal. Proctocolectomy/ileostomy remains the standard procedure for older patients or those with poor continence during acute attacks. Mortality is lower than 2% but ileostomy dysfunction, with an overactive stoma or episodes of obstruction, occurs in about 15% of treated patients.[97]

Subtotal colectomy and ileorectal anastomosis
This is an irrational operation for UC since it leaves the worst affected component of the colon, the rectum, with risks of malignancy developing in the rectal remnant. It has no place in the current surgical management of UC, except in highly selected cases where there is relative rectal sparing and for which **both** pelvic dissection (with a small risk of reduced fertility or impotence) and a stoma need to be avoided. Continuing symptoms are likely. Patients must recognise that this procedure is only a potential surgical bridge until a family is completed and is not a long-term solution.

Ileal pouch–anal anastomosis
"Restorative proctocolectomy" is popular because there is no permanent ileostomy. The entire colon, including the rectum, is removed. The distal 30–40 cm of the ileum is used to create a reservoir (i.e. like the rectum) by anastomosing a variable number of limbs together in a side-to-side fashion before anastomosing this pouch to the anal canal above the dentate line (Figure 9). A temporary ileostomy is usually required for 3–6 months to allow the pouch to heal. The procedure is occasionally performed in one stage (no covering ileostomy), although complications are more serious should they occur. More commonly, it is performed in two stages – colectomy and pouch formation and, later, closure of the covering ileostomy (Figure 9). When an emergency colectomy is performed for severe colitis, or if there is a possibility of Crohn's colitis rather than UC, the procedure is performed in three stages – colectomy and careful histological examination, then pouch formation 3–6 months later, then closure of the ileostomy. There are three different pouch designs (J, S or W) illustrated in Figure 10. Outcomes do not differ, but most surgeons prefer the J pouch.

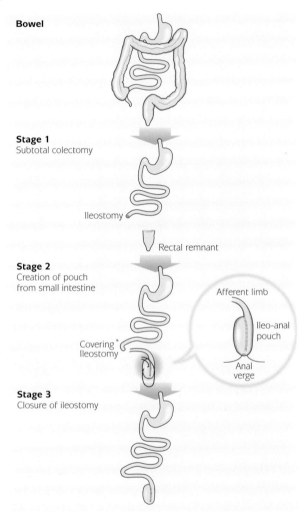

Bowel

Stage 1
Subtotal colectomy

Ileostomy

Rectal remnant

Stage 2
Creation of pouch
from small intestine

Covering
Ileostomy

Afferent limb

Ileo-anal
pouch

Anal
verge

Stage 3
Closure of ileostomy

Figure 9. Creation of an ileo-anal pouch.

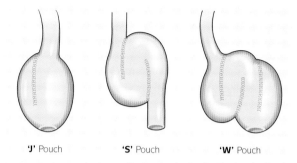

'J' Pouch   'S' Pouch   'W' Pouch

Figure 10. Different ileal pouch designs.

Outcome of ileo-anal pouch surgery

The quality of life is significantly better with an ileo-anal pouch, compared with medical therapy or a permanent ileostomy. In experienced hands, good results (continence and five or fewer bowel actions/day) are obtained in 80–90% of treated patients; 10% have chronic poor function and 5–10% need excision with a permanent ileostomy.[98] A major advantage is the loss of the urgency that characterizes acute colitis, restoring the ability to defer defaecation and to discriminate between flatus and faeces. Medication other than loperamide can be stopped, and the risk of cancer that can complicate extensive colitis is abolished.

Crohn's disease

For CD, surgery should only be undertaken for symptomatic, rather than asymptomatic, radiologically identified disease, because it is potentially panenteric and usually recurs following surgery. Resections should be conservative. Seventy to 80% of patients have an operation at some stage.[99] The decision to operate depends on the degree of disability caused by the symptoms. It is not the aim of this book to review surgical approaches to specific complications, but to highlight the more common procedures.

Indications

Although recurrence is common, surgery should not be delayed when there is a clear indication or medical therapy is failing. Indications are:

- Symptomatic disease despite medical therapy
- Intestinal obstruction (sub-acute or acute) due to strictures
- Local complications (fistula, abscess, perforation).

Small bowel disease

The site of small bowel CD influences the risk of surgery. The data from a tertiary referral centre over a 13-year period showed that 90% patients with ileocolic disease compared with 65% of those with isolated small bowel disease required surgery.[100] The options are resection or stricturoplasty. Stricturoplasy is preferable for small intestinal strictures, since it avoids resection and anastomosis, and minimizes loss of bowel.[101] The anastomotic technique after resection,[102] but not radical resection,[100] may influence recurrence. Bypass procedures should be avoided because the risk of recurrence is high.

Colonic disease

Again, disease anatomy influences the risk of surgery. Almost 75% patients with pancolonic CD need surgery compared with 30% of those with segmental colonic disease. Proctocolectomy remains the gold standard but, unlike UC, may be deferred or avoided by faecal diversion. The advantage of proctocolectomy for isolated colonic disease is that the risk of small bowel disease is very low (< 10% at 15 years), unless there has been previous small bowel involvement. This is not the case with ileocolic disease (clinical recurrence up to 50% at 5 years). Postoperative complications after proctocolectomy are nevertheless common (Table 12), with up to one-third having delayed perineal wound healing and up to 15% with partial erectile dysfunction; up to 20% of those with associated perineal disease require further surgery.

Faecal diversion – by split ileostomy, leaving the colon *in situ* – achieves remission in nearly 90% of patients with colonic disease refractory to medical therapy. Although 45% (or more if there is associated perianal disease) will relapse once the ileostomy is closed, faecal diversion allows time for a patient to come to terms physically and psychologically with an ileostomy.[103] Ileorectal anastomosis may avoid a permanent ileostomy if the rectum is spared, but the relapse rate is higher than with a proctocolectomy. Most surgeons consider ileo-anal pouch formation to be absolutely contraindicated because of the risk of postoperative sepsis or fistulae.

Reducing the risk of postoperative relapse in Crohn's disease

Stop smoking

For those who smoke, stopping smoking significantly reduces postoperative relapse.[103;104] All smokers should be strongly advised to stop, with help offered to achieve this.

Mesalazine after small bowel resection

Mesalazine (3 g/day) lowers postoperative recurrence after small bowel resection (22% *vs* 40% for placebo), but is ineffective after colonic resection.[105] It should normally be given for 18 months.[106]

Azathioprine for complex disease

AZA (1.5–2.5 mg/kg/day) or MP (0.75–1.5mg/kg/day) prevents postoperative recurrence and appears to be better than mesalazine. In 131 patients after ileal or ileocolic resection, the clinical relapse rate at 2 years was 53% on MP (50 mg/day), compared with 61% on mesalazine (3 g/day) and 70% on placebo.[107] AZA is appropriate if disease has frequently relapsed prior to surgery, or after surgery for fistulating disease or a second operation.[108]

Clinical problem: managing a patient with an ileo-anal pouch

It is normal for patients with an ileo-anal pouch to evacuate three to five times a day, and perhaps once at night, but with complete continence and without urgency. It helps to document five objective measures of current function: diurnal and nocturnal frequency, urgency, and diurnal and nocturnal continence. Loperamide, or other antidiarrhoeal agents, may be necessary to achieve optimum function. Pouch dysfunction is the province of specialists, and all patients with a pouch should have long-term specialist follow-up. Stomatherapists (in the department of colorectal surgery) provide a valuable source of information.

Problems with pouches

Stool cultures should be obtained for patients who present with increased pouch frequency, or bleeding, to exclude the possibility of infection, and examination of the mucosa ("pouchoscopy" with a standard sigmoidoscope) should be performed. The main causes of increased pouch frequency are summarized in Table 13.

Pouchitis occurs in up to 45% of patients 5 years after pouch surgery. The cause is unknown, but most have an isolated episode. It is a "new" disease characterized by increased pouch frequency, with or without bleeding, and with mucosal inflammation documented by pouchoscopy and mucosal biopsy. Few trials of treatment have been conducted.[109] Metronidazole (400 mg three times/day) or ciprofloxacin (250 mg twice/day) for 2 weeks are first-line

---

Table 13. Main causes of increased pouch frequency

Increased frequency may be due to:
- Infection
- Pouchitis
- Partial small bowel obstruction
- Cuffitis
- Pelvic sepsis
- Peri-pouch inflammation
- Irritable pouch

therapy. Long-term low-dose metronidazole, or ciprofloxacin, is potentially effective for chronic pouchitis. VSL3 (a commercial mixture of eight different bacterial species) probiotic therapy, although not widely available, is effective for chronic pouchitis at the dose of two sachets, three times daily.[110]

Less common conditions (cuffitis, due to a rim of retained rectal mucosa at the ileopouch–anal anastomosis), pelvic sepsis or an irritable pouch also cause symptoms similar to those of pouchitis.

Complications of inflammatory bowel diseases

Fistulae and abscess formation in Crohn's disease

Abscesses or fistulae occur in up to one-third of patients with CD.[111] A fissuring ulcer first develops, followed by an abscess and then a fistula as the abscess discharges and connects to another epithelial surface (Figure 11). Although uncomplicated perianal disease (simple fissure or fistula-in-ano) can occur in UC, recurrent abscesses or complex fistulae always suggests CD.

Clinical features

Clinical features are classically those of sepsis: severe pain, fever and malaise. Most are perianal. Abdominal entero-cutaneous fistulae most commonly complicate previous

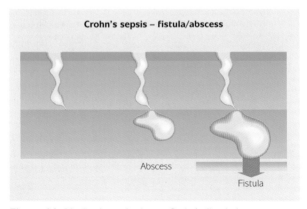

Figure 11. Mechanism of primary Crohn's fistulation: formation of fissuring ulcer, followed by abscess cavity and through fistula. Reproduced with permission from West R, Scott NA. Abdominal fistulizing Crohn's disease. In: Inflammatory bowel diseases, edited by J Satsangi and LR Sutherland. Edinburgh: Churchill Livingstone. 2003.

surgery. CD (usually ileal, occasionally sigmoid colon) can, however, cause a spontaneous psoas or pelvic abscess that later fistulates. Key components of management are to define the anatomy, drain sepsis, control infection, support nutrition, treat active disease and delay relapse. Treatment is complex since recurrence is common, and referral to a specialist centre is often appropriate for management of enterocutaneous fistulae.

Defining anatomy

For perianal disease, pelvic MR is the procedure of choice. It identifies any complex internal fistulation and complements examination under anaesthetic.[112] For abdominal or pelvic collections, a combination of computed tomography (CT) scan, contrast radiology (of the small bowel or colon) and MR are needed prior to surgery.

Initial management

For perianal abscess or fistulae, prompt referral to colorectal surgeons or joint IBD clinic is appropriate. Metronidazole (400 mg three times/day) can be started, but this does not replace drainage, and one or more "seton" is inserted for fistulae. A seton is a loop of monofilament nylon that is inserted along the fistula and tied loosely to prevent distal ends of the fistula closing and forming a recurrent abscess (Figure 12). It is an adjunct to medical treatment and usually stays in place for months. The management of abdominal enterocutaneous fistulae is beyond the scope of this book, where only an outline of the principles is provided (see earlier). Good nutrition is fundamental and may be enteral or parenteral for months before definitive surgery. Neglecting nutrition results in recurrent fistulae.

Subsequent management

Simple perianal fistulae (defined on MR as a single track, below the levator ani) may need no further treatment, but a high proportion will recur. Seton drainage with AZA (see *Surgical therapy in inflammatory bowel disease – Reducing*

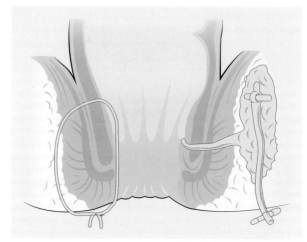

Figure 12. Management of perianal fistulae – sagittal view of the perianal region showing a seton drain in place (left) and catheter drainage of the ischiorectal fossa (right). Reproduced with permission from Judge TA, Lichtenstein GR. Fistulizing Crohn's disease. In: Kirsner's inflammatory bowel diseases, edited by R Balfour Sartor and WJ Sandborn. Edinburgh: Saunders. 2004.

the risk of postoperative relapse in Crohn's disease; Azathioprine for complex disease) to delay recurrence and intermittent metronidazole for active sepsis provides adequate control. IFX provides short-term benefit (*see Medical therapy – Infliximab*), but in the UK it is not approved by NICE for this indication. For complex fistulae (branching track or above the levator ani), colonoscopy to reassess disease activity after drainage and seton insertion are appropriate. Active disease is treated with steroids (or more effectively by IFX if severe) as long as any abscess has been excluded by clinical and radiological examination. AZA should be started and a joint decision made between the gastroenterologist and colorectal surgeon about the timing of removal of the seton(s). Faecal diversion by colostomy (if there is no proximal colonic disease) or ileostomy is occasionally necessary for severe perianal disease, especially if a stricture has developed or continence impaired. Other medical therapies, such as long term antibiotics, enteral nutriton to "medically" defunction the colon or tacrolimus, belong to the province of specialists.

Osteoporosis

Osteoporosis is common in patients with inflammatory bowel, although the absolute fracture risk is small and the role of prophylaxis remains debated. Diagnosis is best made by dual energy x-ray absorptiometry (DXA) bone scan, judged by the T-score (standard deviations in relation to peak bone mass; *see* Table 14).

Risk of fracture

In a population-based study of 238 patients with CD diagnosed between 1940 and 1993, 63 had 117 different fractures, with a cumulative incidence of 36% at 20 years, compared with 32% in controls (odds ratio 0.9; 95% confidence interval 0.6–1.4; $P = 0.79$).[113] Neither corticosteroid nor surgical resection was predictor of fracture risk. Only age emerged as a significant predictor (hazard ratio 1.3 per decade; 95% confidence interval 1.1–1.5). A single study examined the relationship between low bone mineral density and prevalence of vertebral fractures.[114] In 271 patients with ileocaecal CD, asymptomatic fractures were observed on lumbar spine x-ray in 25 out of 179 (14%) steroid-free patients and 13 out of 89 (15%) steroid-dependent patients. The fracture rate in steroid-naive patients was 12%, and did not correlate with bone mineral density. However, a British study of 231,778 fracture cases compared with 231,778 age- and sex-matched controls found a 72% increase in vertebral

Table 14. T-scores for the diagnosis of osteoporosis	
> -1	Normal
-1 to -2.5	Osteopenia
< -2.5	Osteoporosis

fractures and 59% increase in hip fractures in those who had IBD, compared with those who did not have this condition.[115]

General measures
All patients should be encouraged to exercise,[116] have an adequate calcium intake (using supplements if restricting dairy intake) and avoid smoking (Table 15).

Treatment
Bisphosphonates and hormone replacement therapy have been tried in CD and UC. In 32 patients with CD with a T-score of inferior to -1, alendronate (10 mg/day) increased vertebral bone mineral density by 5.5% compared with placebo ($P = 0.01$).[117] In 47 postmenopausal women with IBD, hormone replacement therapy increased vertebral bone mineral density by +2.6% at 1 year, but this trial lacked controls.[118]

Indications for DXA scan
Patients who have been on steroids for more than 3 months in a year are best offered a DXA scan. Some advocate a scan at diagnosis and at arbitrary 5-year intervals, or if there is a strong family history of osteoporosis, but there is no evidence to support this.

Indications for treatment
Patients with a vertebral or hip T-score inferior to -1.5, those who develop a fragility fracture or those who are taking long-term steroids are reasonably offered bisphosphonates (alendronate 70 mg once/week, or risendronate 35 mg once/week).

Table 15. General measures for the prevention of osteoporosis associated with inflammatory bowel disease

Minimum dose of glucocorticoids
Regular exercise
Lifestyle modifications (stop smoking, reduce alcohol)
Calcium/vitamin D supplementation
Correct malnutrition

Colorectal cancer

The risk of colorectal cancer is increased for those patients with UC or CD with long-standing (> 10 years), extensive (proximal to the splenic flexure) colitis, but the value of surveillance colonoscopy remains debated. It is important to discuss with individual patients their risk of colorectal cancer, the implications should dysplasia be identified, the limitations of surveillance (which may miss dysplasia) and the small, but definable, risks of colonoscopy. A joint decision on the appropriateness of surveillance can then be made, taking the patient's views into account. A practical approach is described in Figure 13.

Actual risk

Early studies overestimated risk, because they came from referral centres with a higher proportion of patients with extensive or chronic active disease. In a meta-analysis of 116 studies, the cumulative incidence in UC was 2% by 10 years, 8% by 20 years and 18% by 30 years.[119] However, there were only 13 population-based studies, and in a Danish cohort of 1,161 patients with UC the cancer risk was no different from that of the general population.[120] This may reflect the high colectomy rate (32%) in this population. The risk of colorectal cancer in colonic CD is considered similar to UC of similar extent and duration.[121]

Risk factors

The risk factors for colorectal cancer in ulcerative colitis are shown in Table 16, and disease extent is the most important of these factors. In a population-based cohort of 3,117 patients, proctitis did not increase the risk, while the risk in left-sided colitis was 2.8 (confidence interrval 1.6– 4.4) and 14.8 in pancolitis (11.4–18.9).122 Lennard-Jones *et al.* looked prospectively at 401 UC patients with extensive disease over 22 years,[123] and found that the cumulative probability of developing colorectal cancer was 3% at 15 years, 5% at 20 years and 9% at 25 years. These findings confirm the importance of disease duration as a risk factor. Young age at

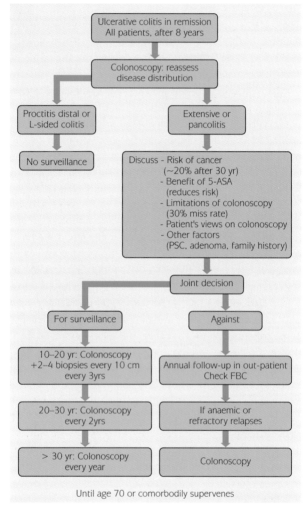

Figure 13. Practical approach to surveillance colonoscopy
(5-ASA = 5-aminosalicylates; PSC = primary sclerosing
cholangitis; FBC = full blood count).

Table 16. Risk factors for colorectal cancer in ulcerative colitis

Key factors
Disease extent (extensive or pancolitis)
Disease duration (>10 years)
Primary sclerosing cholangitis

Indirect risk factors
Age at onset of disease
Family history of cancer
Co-existent adenoma

Risk modifiers
Sulfasalazine/mesalazine

onset increases the duration of exposure (cancers may develop at a younger age), but does not otherwise increase the risk. PSC is infrequent (2–4% of UC), but substantially increases the risk (by 33% at 20 years) of colorectal cancer.[124] Maintenance therapy with sulfasalazine or mesalazine decreases the risk by up to 90% (odds ratio 0.09; confidence interval 0.03–0.28 for mesalazine at 1.2g/day or more).[119] This should be a major inducement for continuing maintenance therapy.

Anaemia

Anaemia often complicates IBD. One-third of patients will have a Hb level lower than 12 g/dl, with an associated reduction in quality of life, cognitive function and working capacity (Figure 14). Anaemia is too often neglected as an inevitable component of UC or CD, when it may often be corrected.[125]

Assessment

The initial step is to perform haematinics (ferritin, folate and B_{12} assay). Iron deficiency is most common, due to overt or occult blood loss or dietary restriction, but vitamin B_{12} deficiency in CD (ileal disease, or > 100 cm terminal ileal resection), folate deficiency (proximal intestinal CD or dietary restriction), haemolysis (rarely associated with UC or CD, or

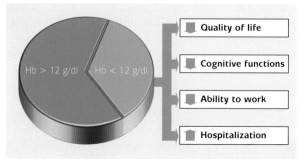

Figure 14. Anaemia complications in inflammatory bowel disease, and their socio-economic impact. Reproduced with permission from Gasche C. Anemia in inflammatory bowel disease. In: Inflammatory bowel diseases, edited by J Satsangi and LR Sutherland. Edinburgh: Churchill Livingstone. 2003.

due to drugs) and bone-marrow suppression (usually due to drugs) also occur. Ferritin, a measure of iron stores, is an acute-phase reactant and so may be elevated during active disease even if iron deficiency exists; a concentration less than 55 µg/l makes marrow iron depletion likely.[126] A new iron index – serum transferring-receptor concentrations in combination with serum ferritin – helps identify iron deficiency more accurately and predicts response to intravenous iron therapy.[127] The new development of iron deficiency in UC is an indication for colonoscopy to exclude a complicating carcinoma. Refractory iron deficiency in UC or CD may be due to associated coeliac disease.

Management

Oral iron therapy is often poorly tolerated, making replacement difficult. This may be because ferric ions contribute to active inflammation. Nevertheless, for those with modest iron-deficiency anaemia (Hb 10.0–12.0 g/dl), oral iron should be tried. There is no objective evidence that any one preparation (ferrous sulphate, gluconate or fumarate) is any better or worse tolerated than another. Beware of "over the counter" preparations, especially those with "added vitamins": these often contain smaller doses of iron (as little as 9 mg/tablet) to improve tolerability. Elemental iron (200 mg/day)for 3 months is needed to replace iron stores.

Intravenous iron

For more severe anaemia (Hb < 10g/dl), or the 25% of individuals who cannot tolerate oral iron, intravenous iron is appropriate. Intravenous iron dextran (Imferon) had a bad reputation for anaphylaxis. Iron sucrose (Venofer) is safer, but needs to be given several times over a 2-week period to replace iron stores. The dose is calculated from the Hb level and body weight. A new form of iron dextran (CosmoFer) appears to be safe, and allows a single total dose of iron infusion over 4 hours to be administered as a day case. Intramuscular iron sorbitol (Jectofer) has been withdrawn from the UK. Supraphysiologic doses of erythropoietin have been shown to be effective in refractory anaemia of chronic disease,[128] because this hormone overcomes cytokine-induced inhibition of erythropoeisis. It is expensive and its role is limited. Gastroenterologists need to be more aware about the impact of under-treated anaemia and may need prompting from primary care.

Clinical problem: which patients need cancer surveillance?

UK guidelines advise that patients with UC should have a colonoscopy after 8–10 years to re-evaluate disease extent.[129]

Selection

Surveillance is only appropriate for patients with extensive colitis. It is not known whether patients with previously extensive disease and whose disease has regressed benefit from surveillance. For those with extensive colitis opting for surveillance, colonoscopies should be conducted every 3 years in the second decade, every 2 years in the third decade, and annually in the fourth decade of disease. Four random biopsies every 10 cm from the entire colon are best taken with additional samples of suspicious areas. Patients with PSC should have more frequent, perhaps annual, colonoscopy. Evidence in support of this approach is circumstantial.

Problems with colonoscopy surveillance

Patients and their doctors should understand that colonoscopic surveillance may miss cancers or dysplasia in up to 30% of cases. They should also understand that the purpose of surveillance is to detect dysplasia or cancer at an early stage, with a view to colectomy. It is estimated that 56 biopsies are needed to exclude dysplasia with 95% confidence, and 33 biopsies with 90% confidence. Most surveillance procedures achieve less than 20 biopsies. Furthermore, dysplasia is open to interpretation, and agreement about the diagnosis of low-grade dysplasia between specialist pathologists is about 70%.[130] Furthermore, over 100 colonoscopies have to be performed to detect one case of dysplasia or cancer. Add to this the small, but real, risk of perforation or haemorrhage during colonoscopy (1:1000 per procedure – equivalent to 1:250 for four procedures), then some patients may elect to take an expectant approach. There is no value in surveillance if concomitant illness or advanced age makes colectomy inappropriate.

Options other than colonoscopic surveillance

In one UK region, those patients with extensive colitis who defaulted from specialist follow-up had the highest number of cancers.[131] A practical option is to conduct at least an annual follow-up of patients with extensive colitis, continued maintenance therapy, and prompt colonoscopy in the event of anaemia or recurrent symptoms that do not rapidly respond to treatment. The doctor should help the patient make an informed choice.

Inflammatory bowel diseases in pregnancy, children and adolescents

Fertility

Male fertility

Up to 10% of couples within the normal population will experience problems with fertility.[132] Table 17 summarizes male infertility in IBD. Male patients with UC or CD have normal fertility, except those on sulfasalazine (unlike other 5-ASAs), which causes oligospermia in more than 50% of treated patients. This is usually reversible within 2 months after stopping the medication.[133] Immunomodulators such as AZA or MP also reduce sperms counts compared with controls, but not below the normal range, and parameters of sperm quality remain within World Health Organization normal values.[134] One study examined the outcome of pregnancy when fathers were treated with AZA or MP for IBD.[63;135] There were 154 pregnancies from 76 male patients (each patient fathering one to six pregnancies; median = 2).There were no differences in spontaneous abortion, congenital abnormalities or neoplasia compared with patients who had fathered children before AZA or MP was started.

Female fertility

Women with UC or CD have fewer offspring than similarly age matched controls from the general population.[132] This may reflect factors such as relationship difficulties, incorrect perceptions of pregnancy with IBD or simply personal choice. Table 17 summarizes female infertility in IBD. Women with CD have reduced fertility during active disease, but have otherwise normal fertility during quiescent disease. Consequently, control of active disease should be a priority in patients that wish to have children.[136] This also applies to UC with one important exception: patients who have

Table 17. Male and female fertility in inflammatory bowel disease	
Male fertility	**Female fertility**

• Normal sperm count, except:
  - Oligospermia caused by sulfasalazine reversible upon cessation of treatment
  - Reduced sperm count by azathioprine/mercaptopurine but not below WHO normal values
	• Reduced fertility during active disease
	• Conception better deferred until remission
	• Lower fertility after pelvic dissection compared with ileostomy or medical therapy*

*See Management during pregnancy

undergone pelvic dissection (during ileo-anal pouch surgery or proctocolectomy) have lower fertility than that of comparable patients with an ileostomy or who are maintained on medical therapy. In 237 women who had had an ileo-anal pouch for UC, the number of births from disease onset to colectomy was not significantly decreased (120 compared with 131 expected), but in the 12 months after ileostomy closure only 34 deliveries occurred compared with 69 that were expected ($P < 0.001$).[137] The effect of AZA and other medication is discussed later in this section. In general, women, including those seeking *in vitro* fertilization, should be advised to defer conception until remission.

Efficacy of contraceptives in inflammatory bowel diseases
Theoretical risks of poor absorption of oral contraceptives in patients with small intestinal CD and diarrhoea, ileostomy or ileo-anal pouch for UC should be discussed with the patient. Evidence of impaired effect is lacking, but "mini pills" should perhaps be used with caution.

Management during pregnancy
Risk of relapse
Pregnant women with UC or CD have no increased risk of relapse during pregnancy. About one-third of these patients report improvement, one-third describes no change and one-third deteriorates during pregnancy. However, if disease is active at conception, then at least 50% continue to relapse.[138]

Population-based studies have shown no increased risk of stillbirth, and no neonatal complications or congenital anomalies, although a tendency to low birth weight and preterm delivery has been reported.[139-141]

Medical treatment during pregnancy

The aim should be to maintain remission by continuing maintenance therapy during pregnancy. The risk of active disease to the foetus is higher than theoretical risks of drugs commonly used to maintain remission. The safety of IBD medications during pregnancy is summarized in Table 18.

Table 18. Safety of drugs used for inflammatory bowel diseases during pregnancy	
Benefit of remission outweighs risk	**Not recommended**
Aminosalicylates (< 3 g/day: no increased risk of birth defects) Corticosteroids Azathioprine/mercaptopurine Metronidazole (short courses)	Ciprofloxacin/other fluoroquinolones Methotrexate ? Ciclosporin ? Infliximab

5-Aminosalicylates in pregnancy

For 5-ASA, mothers can be advised that, although small amounts of 5-ASA and its metabolite can be detected in cord blood during treatment, multiple studies have shown that 5-ASA below 3 g/day does not increase the risk of birth defects. In 165 patients treated with 5-SA during pregnancy, major malformations occurred in 0.8% of patients on 5-ASA and in 3.8% in controls. There was an increase in preterm deliveries (13.0% *vs* 4.7%) and, consequently, a slightly lower birth weight (mean 3252 *vs* 3461 g); however, the benefit of maintaining remission balanced the risk.[142]

Steroids in pregnancy

Corticosteroids can be used in exactly the same way as non-pregnant women; indeed there is more danger from under-treated active disease than from steroids. Placental enzymes metabolize 90% of the maternal dose.[143]

Azathioprine or mercaptopurine in pregnancy

Thiopurines also appear to be safe. In 171 pregnancies in 75 women treated with MP in New York, the relative risk of spontaneous abortion, congenital anomaly or puerperal infection was 0.85 (confidence interval 0.47–1.55; $P = 0.59$).[63]

Other drugs for inflammatory bowel diseases

Ciprofloxacin, and other fluoroquinolones, may cause an arthropathy and should be avoided. Short courses of metronidazole are safe. Methotrexate, a known teratogen, should be avoided or used with considerable caution in women of childbearing age.[144] IFX has been coincidentally given in pregnancy, with 26 live births out of 35, and five spontaneous and four therapeutic abortions.[145] It cannot be recommended, although there is no need for therapeutic termination if coincidental administration occurs.

Delivery

Normal delivery is possible and appropriate, with the exception of patients with perineal CD or an ileo-anal pouch. While normal delivery has often been reported in both conditions, the obstetric complications can have such major impact that patients are usually best advised to have a caesarian section. Rectovaginal fistula can occur after episiotomy in perineal CD, and any disruption of anal sphincter function in a patient with an ileo-anal pouch may cause impaired faecal continence. These issues should be discussed with the patient.

Breastfeeding

Nearly all drugs used to treat UC or CD are secreted in breast milk. A balance has to be struck between the benefits of breastfeeding and risk of small amounts of the drug to the baby. Inevitably, there are few data. For prednisolone, less than 0.1% of the oral dose appears in breast milk, equivalent to less than 10% of foetal cortisol production.[146] AZA is more contentious, because of the theoretical risk of immune suppression, and bottle-feeding or stopping AZA, having discussed risks of relapse (*see Medical therapy – Immunomodulatory therapy*), is usually recommended.

Children and adolescents

Management of children with UC or CD should best be through a tertiary centre with a paediatric gastroenterologist. Unique to paediatric populations are the implications of the disease on growth, development and education (Table 19).

Table 19. Important issues in therapeutic strategy for children with inflammatory bowel disease

- Disease location
- Patient's growth (current centile chart)
- Patient's growth rate
- Nutritional status and body mass index
- Stage of puberty
- Bone age (measure of growth potential)
- Social history, family dynamics and school performance

Clinical features

Both UC and CD have similar features to those in adults, although CD may more commonly affect the small bowel[147] and UC may be more extensive.[148;149]

Growth retardation

Impairment of linear growth in CD precedes diagnosis in 50% of cases, and continues in the first years after diagnosis, although this is uncommon (10%) in UC.[150] Despite this, more than two-thirds of adolescents with CD will reach their normal predicted adult height.[151] Height velocity correlates with disease activity, and the most important message is that weight **and** height are recorded on appropriate centile charts at each clinic visit.

Development

Pubertal delay is common, again more often in CD than UC. Chronic under nutrition is the principal cause and also accounts for most growth retardation.

Management differences to adults

Key differences from adult management are that primary enteral nutrition is first-line treatment for small intestinal CD, growth retardation is an indication for surgical intervention and AZA may be considered for primary prophylaxis.

Nutritional therapy

In 78 children with small bowel CD randomized to either enteral therapy or corticosteroids, 75% in the group given enteral nutrition responded to treatment, compared with 89% in the group given alternate-day corticosteroids.[152] Growth and weight gain were, however, higher in the enteral nutrition group.[152] Nocturnal nasogastric feeding may be necessary, but compliance is better in children than in adults and the main value of feeding is to reverse undernutriton in active disease. There is no place for enteral feeding as treatment for paediatric UC.

Azathioprine in children

Primary prophylaxis with MP (1 mg/kg) for 12 months after diagnosis of CD resulted in better growth, lower cumulative dose of steroids and fewer relapses in a prospective, placebo-controlled trial.[153] It is safe and in combination with nutritional therapy and can be extremely effective.[154]

Timing of surgery

Surgical indications in IBD are similar to adults, with the exception that surgery (resection for CD or colectomy for UC) is appropriate if growth retardation does not resolve within months on medical therapy. Delay has long-term consequences if epiphyses fuse. Timing is crucial, taking into account the school year, nutritional status and growth potential.

From the time of diagnosis, it is important that an atmosphere is created in which both children and parents, together or independently, can express their concerns about physical and psychological aspects of the disease (Table 20).

Table 20. Key concerns in 117 children with inflammatory disease from Canada*†

Bothered by having to take medicines
Worried about the possibility of having a flare-up
Upset that inflammatory bowel disease is a life-long condition
Concerned about weight
Worried about health problems in the future
Bothered about height
Bothered about stomach pains/cramps
Inability/not enough energy to perform certain activities
Unfair to have bowel disease
Stomach pains/cramps
Tiredness
Frustration
Concerned/upset by physical appearance resulting from bowel disease
Worried about needing surgery

*In order of importance.
†From Richardson G, Griffiths AM, Miller V, Thomas AG. Quality of life in inflammatory bowel disease: a cross-cultural comparison of English and Canadian children. *J Pediatr J Gastroenterol Nutr* 2001;**32**:573–578.

A multidisciplinary team involving the paediatric nurse specialist, dietician, and specific surgeon and psychologist is crucial to achieve this. Support in coping with a chronic illness and achieving maximum educational potential must be provided.

Clinical problem: family history and risk of inflammatory bowel diseases

The risk of IBD to the children's sibling or other relatives is the cause for much anxiety to patients and their families. In 640 patients with IBD in Belgium, 5% had an affected sibling, 2% an affected parent and 7% an affected child. Overall, the percentage of first-degree relatives affected was 4%.[155] The simplest message is that, while children of an affected parent are at higher risk, they have more than 90% chance of **not** being affected. In a nation-wide study from Denmark, the risk of UC or CD among children of patients with IBD was two to13 times higher than that of the general population.[156] When both parents are affected by IBD, the risk is higher,[157] but numbers are too small to make reliable estimates.

Inflammatory bowel disease

Prognosis

The prognosis of IBD is summarized in Table 21.

Table 21. Prognosis in inflammatory disease				
Condition	Prognosis after 1 year	Prognosis on maintenance of therapy	Mortality	Employability
Ulcerative colitis	Intermittent activity in 90% patients Remission in 50% patients Relapse in 20% patients every year	Remission in 50–60% patients for > 2 years No symptoms in < 5% patients for 15 years	Same as in general population, except pancolitis in first 2 years after diagnosis (especially if > 50 years old at diagnosis)	~ 90% patients fully capable of work after 1st year of diagnosis
Crohn's disease			Slightly higher than in normal population Higher than in ulcerative colitis	75% patients fully capable of work in 1st year after diagnosis 15% patients unable to work after 5–10 years of disease

Course of ulcerative colitis

The pattern of relapse and remission 1 year after diagnosis of UC tends to continue for any individual. Ninety per cent of patients have intermittent activity, and 50% are in remission at any one time. Twenty per cent relapse every year, and 10% have continuous symptoms. Prolonged remission on maintenance therapy occurs, with 50–60% of patients remaining in remission for more than 2 years, but fewer than 5% are symptom-free for 15 years. Colectomy rate varies with the local approach to refractory disease, between 11 and 32%.

Course of Crohn's disease

The course of CD in any given patient cannot be predicted. Relapses tend to follow the previous pattern of disease (fibrostenotic, fistulating, inflammatory). Up to 80% concordance of disease distribution or pattern has been reported in family members affected by CD. Most patients have a good prognosis, although morbidity may be considerable for short periods. CD cannot be cured, but a year after diagnosis, about 50% of patients have no symptoms, 25% have low activity, and 25% high-disease activity in any given year.

Mortality in ulcerative colitis

The overall mortality for UC is similar to that in the general population, with the exception of patients with pancolitis in the first 2 years after diagnosis, especially if the patient is older than 50 years at diagnosis.

Evidence

Of 261 deaths in a cohort of 1,160 patients followed for a median of 19 (range 1–36) years, only 10% were attributable to complications of UC. Twenty-three out of 25 deaths due to UC were in patients who had extensive colitis and a median age of 62 at diagnosis.[158] Although these results were from a population-based study, they were from a single specialist centre and should be compared with those from a large cohort study, which examined IBD-related mortality in the UK.[159] This study conducted on the records from the UK General Practice Research Database found 536 deaths in 8,301 patients with UC. When these deaths were compared with 2,096 deaths in 41,589 matched controls, UC-related mortality was found to be 44% (odds ratio 1.44; confidence interval 1.31–1.58), a much higher proportion than that found in the other study. Although the large cohort study reflected variations in regional practice more accurately, a correlation between mortality and disease extent could not be established.

Mortality in Crohn's disease

The overall mortality of CD is slightly higher than that in the normal population, and is higher than that of UC. It is greatest in the 2 years after diagnosis or in patients with upper gastrointestinal disease.

Evidence

In the large cohort study using records from the General Practice Research Database (mentioned earlier), 351 deaths in 5,960 cases of CD were compared with 1,095 deaths in 29,843 controls.[159] Excess mortality was found to be 73% (odds ratio 1.73; confidence interval 1.54–1.96). To put this in perspective: this increase in mortality is of the same order of magnitude as the increase in standardized mortality ratio in healthy individuals by many occupations.

Employability

After the first year of disease, approximately 90% of patients are fully capable of work (defined by < 1 month off work/year), although UC causes significant employment problems in a minority of patients. CD tends to cause greater disability than UC, with only 75% of patients fully capable of work in the year after diagnosis and 15% of patients unable to work after 5–10 years of disease.

Frequently asked questions

What is inflammatory bowel disease?

"Inflammatory bowel disease"' is a general term for two causes of inflammation in the gut, called ulcerative colitis and Crohn's disease, when the intestines become inflamed and ulcerated. Symptoms can include diarrhoea (sometimes with blood and mucus), pain in the abdomen, weight loss and tiredness. Both conditions are characterized by unpredictable episodes of relapse, when symptoms occur, and periods of remission, when the person feels well. Inflammatory bowel disease (IBD) is quite different from irritable bowel syndrome (IBS).

What are the differences between Crohn's disease and Ulcerative colitis?

Area affected

Ulcerative colitis only affects the colon (large intestine). When it only affects the rectum, it is known as proctitis. In Crohn's disease, the affected area may cover the small intestine as well as the colon (30% affects the small intestine alone, 30% the colon alone and 30% both the small intestine and colon). The mouth, anus or other areas of the digestive system can also be affected (10%).

Inflammation

In ulcerative colitis, only the inner surface lining of the colon (the mucosa) is inflamed, whereas in Crohn's disease, all layers of the bowel may be inflamed.

Common symptoms

In ulcerative colitis, the most common symptom is bloody diarrhoea. Pain in the abdomen is usually absent, or moderate, rather than severe. In Crohn's disease, diarrhoea (often with little blood), abdominal pain that may be severe and weight loss are the common symptoms.

Complications

Complications in ulcerative colitis are anaemia and, in severe colitis, dilatation of the colon; those in Crohn's disease are intestinal abscess, obstruction and fistulae (abnormal passages).

Treatment

Treatment for ulcerative colitis includes steroids for acute attacks, and mesalazine or azathioprine to prevent relapse. For Crohn's disease, treatment includes steroids, liquid diet or mesalazine for acute attacks, and mesalazine or azathioprine to prevent relapse.

How common are ulcerative colitis and Crohn's disease ?

Between 150,000 and 250,000 people are affected by ulcerative colitis or Crohn's disease in the UK – that's about 1 in 500. The illnesses can start at any age, but most commonly between the ages of 15 and 40 years.

What causes ulcerative colitis or Crohn's disease?

The cause(s) of neither ulcerative colitis nor Crohn's disease is known, but the consensus is that the immune system is triggered by unknown ("environmental") factors in genetically susceptible individuals. One gene (the NOD2 gene) has been found, which accounts for about a third of Crohn's disease in the small intestine. Genes for ulcerative colitis have not yet been found. "Environmental" factors that could trigger the immune system are likely to include bacteria usually present in the gut, or an unusual response to a common infection. Once triggered, the immune system over-reacts to cause the inflammation and ulceration in the intestine. Drugs to treat IBD are primarily designed to damp down this overactive immune response.

Is there a connection between the measles/mumps/rubella (MMR) vaccine and IBD ?

Despite an early report suggesting that there may be a link to Crohn's disease, almost everyone (including some of the authors of the original report) now agrees that there is *no excess risk* of developing Crohn's disease (or ulcerative colitis) after vaccination with MMR.

Does smoking affect IBD?

Smoking has different effects on ulcerative colitis and Crohn's disease. Ulcerative colitis is most likely to occur in ex-smokers or non-smokers – and one of very few diseases that is *less* likely to occur in smokers. If ulcerative colitis starts, however, starting smoking does not help and has so many other unwelcome effects that it cannot be advised.

In contrast, smoking makes Crohn's disease *more likely*. Furthermore, continuing to smoke in Crohn's disease increases the risk of relapse, need for steroids and need for surgery.

My mother has IBD – what are my chances of developing it?

A mother (like a child) is a "first-degree relative", and the risk of developing ulcerative colitis or Crohn's in the child of a parent with IBD is about 5% (1 in 20). That's a 95% chance of *not* developing the condition. The risk is higher if two first-degree relatives are affected.

Is there a risk of cancer with IBD?

Most people with ulcerative colitis only have a small proportion of their colon affected, and the risk of developing cancer of the colon is *no greater* than normal (the normal life time risk is 2–3%). In the proportion of people whose whole colon is affected, however, the risk of colon cancer is increased, depending on the duration of symptoms. The risk only starts to increase after 10 years and, by 30 years, about 20% of patients who have ulcerative colitis affecting the whole colon will develop colon cancer. The good news is that regular preventive treatment with sulfasalazine or 5-aminisaalicylates appears to decrease the risk.

In Crohn's disease, only a very small proportion of people have Crohn's colitis affecting the whole colon after 10 years but, in these people, the risk of colon cancer is also increased by the same degree. The risk of small bowel cancer is probably also increased in people when Crohn's affects the small intestine, but small bowel cancer is so very rare that it remains very rare.

Is surveillance colonoscopy necessary for IBD?

The simple answer is that not everyone needs regular colonoscopy. "Surveillance" means that the purpose of colonoscopy is to pick up warning signs of cancer when there are no symptoms. This only needs to be considered in people with ulcerative colitis, whose whole colon is affected and who have had symptoms for 10 years or more – that's less than 1 in 5 of all people with ulcerative colitis. Although colonoscopy is currently the best way of picking up early signs of cancer, it is still not very good. Up to 30% of warning signs may not be detected and it carries a small risk as well as being unpleasant. Consequently, the pros and cons of surveillance should be carefully discussed between the patient and specialist. Some conditions (such as polyps or the condition of primary sclerosing cholangitis) may increase the risk of cancer, and other things (such as medication) reduce that risk.

Does IBD reduce fertility?

Women with ulcerative colitis should have the same chance of becoming pregnant as women without ulcerative colitis. Men who are taking sulfasalazine as treatment for ulcerative colitis, however, have a reduced sperm count, but this is reversible so this medication is usually changed in men who want to become fathers.

Women and men with Crohn's disease may have reduced fertility, especially during a period of active disease. Some women with Crohn's disease find it difficult to become pregnant, because inflammation around the bowel can affect the fallopian tubes. However, many people with Crohn's disease have children with no trouble at all.

Will my pregnancy be normal if I have IBD?

The key to a healthy pregnancy in somebody with ulcerative colitis or Crohn's disease is to keep the condition in remission and well controlled. The best time to try for a baby is when the IBD is in remission, usually on regular medication. Regular medication with all treatment commonly used in IBD (including mesalazine and azathioprine) is safer for mother and baby than a relapse.

Pregnancy does *not* make either ulcerative colitis or Crohn's disease worse, but stopping regular medication will increase the risk of relapse. Normal delivery is possible, although mothers with Crohn's disease affecting the anus or rectum, or those who have an internal pouch, are usually advised to have a Caesarean section. Breast-feeding is also normally possible, except for people taking some drugs, such as azathioprine or ciprofloxacin.

What is the risk of needing surgery with IBD?

For ulcerative colitis, surgery is effectively a cure (albeit a radical one!) for the condition. The chance of having such troublesome colitis within a lifetime that surgery is necessary is between 10 and 25%, depending on the extent of colitis. Those with extensive colitis have a higher risk. If colitis is severe enough to need admission to hospital for treatment, the chance of colectomy is about 30%.

Most people with Crohn's disease will need an operation at some stage, especially if it affects the small bowel, when 80% need an operation up to 15 years after diagnosis. However, only 10% need more than 2 operations in a lifetime.

Is there a special diet that I should eat?

No food is known to cause ulcerative colitis or Crohn's disease. However, some people find some foods upset them and these foods – if they can be identified – are best avoided. It is important to recognise that not all symptoms of diarrhoea or pain that may occur after eating are due to worsening of the ulcerative colitis or Crohn's disease. Such symptoms are common in people with an irritable bowel (IBS), which may exist as well as IBD.

In general, milk and dairy products are important sources of calcium, and advice to avoid them is commonly wrong. Wheat, tea and coffee, or alcohol, may contribute to wind or looser stools. A well-balanced diet with protein (fish, meat), fat and carbohydrate, with some fruit and vegetable fibre, is usually sensible.

Special diets to exclude fibre are necessary in some people with Crohn's disease who have strictures in the small intestine causing symptoms of obstruction. A liquid diet is also effective for some people, especially children, with active Crohn's disease. If in doubt, diet should be discussed with a qualified dietician at the hospital rather than a self-appointed "nutritionist".

Can you claim disability allowance if you have IBD?

The general answer is "no", unless you are badly affected by ulcerative colitis or Crohn's disease. One of the difficulties for people who assess eligibility for Disability Living Allowance is that people with IBD have variable disability – badly affected during a relapse, but well at other times.

Fortunately, the National Association for Colitis and Crohn's disease in the UK have worked very hard at helping people who think they may be eligible. It is well worth contacting them *before* making an application. Then make sure that the doctor completing the information on the application form has all the key information (continence, bowel frequency, urgency, etc), because it is much easier to get it right first time than to succeed on appeal.

References

1. Farrokhyar F, Swarbrick ET, Irvine EJ. A critical review of epidemiological studies in inflammatory bowel disease. *Scand J Gastroenterol*. 2001;**36**:2-15.

2. Ekbom A, Helmick C, Zack M, Adami HO. The epidemiology of inflammatory bowel disease: a large, population-based study in Sweden. *Gastroenterology* 1991;**100**:350-8.

3. Srivastava ED, Mayberry JF, Morris TJ *et al*. Incidence of ulcerative colitis in Cardiff over 20 years: 1968-87. *Gut* 1992;**33**:256-8.

4. Shivananda S, Lennard-Jones J, Logan R *et al*. Incidence of inflammatory bowel disease across Europe: is there a difference between north and south? Results of the European Collaborative Study on Inflammatory Bowel Disease (EC-IBD). *Gut* 1996;**39**:690-7.

5. Moum B, Vatn MH, Ekbom A *et al*. Incidence of inflammatory bowel disease in southeastern Norway: evaluation of methods after 1 year of registration. Southeastern Norway IBD Study Group of Gastroenterologists. *Digestion* 1995;**56**:377-81.

6. Armitage E, Drummond HE, Wilson DC, Ghosh S. Increasing incidence of both juvenile-onset Crohn's disease and ulcerative colitis in Scotland. *Eur J Gastroenterol Hepatol*. 2001;**13**:1439-47.

7. Munkholm P, Langholz E, Nielsen OH *et al*. Incidence and prevalence of Crohn's disease in the county of Copenhagen, 1962-87: a sixfold increase in incidence. *Scand J Gastroenterol*. 1992;**27**:609-14.

8. Langholz E, Munkholm P, Nielsen OH *et al*. Incidence and prevalence of ulcerative colitis in Copenhagen county from 1962 to 1987. *Scand J Gastroenterol*. 1991;**26**:1247-56.

9. Price AB. Overlap in the spectrum of non-specific inflammatory bowel disease—'colitis indeterminate'. *J Clin Pathol*. 1978;**31**:567-77.

10. Truelove SC, Witts LJ. Cortisone in ulcerative colitis. *BMJ* 1955;**2**:1042-8.

11. Walmsley RS, Ayres RC, Pounder RE *et al*. A simple clinical colitis activity index. *Gut* 1998;**43**:29-32.

12. Harvey RF, Bradshaw JM. A simple index of Crohn's-disease activity. *Lancet* 1980;**1**:514.

13. Salmon JF, Wright JP, Murray AD. Ocular inflammation in Crohn's disease. *Ophthalmology* 1991;**98**:480-4.

14. Bernstein CN, Blanchard JF, Rawsthorne P *et al*. The prevalence of extraintestinal diseases in inflammatory bowel disease: a population-based study. *Am J Gastroenterol*. 2001;**96**:1116-22.

15. Hopkins DJ, Horan E, Burton IL *et al*. Ocular disorders in a series of 332 patients with Crohn's disease. *Br J Ophthalmol*. 1974;**58**:732-7.

16. Orchard TR, Chua CN, Ahmad T *et al*. Uveitis and erythema nodosum in inflammatory bowel disease: clinical features and the role of HLA genes. *Gastroenterology* 2002;**123**:714-8.

17. Mir-Madjlessi SH, Taylor JS, Farmer RG. Clinical course and evolution of erythema nodosum and pyoderma gangrenosum in chronic ulcerative colitis: a study of 42 patients. *Am J Gastroenterol*. 1985;**80**:615-20.

18. Tromm A, May D, Almus E *et al*. Cutaneous manifestations in inflammatory bowel disease. *Z Gastroenterol*. 2001;**39**:137-44.

19. Triantafillidis JK, Cheracakis P, Sklavaina M *et al*. Favorable response to infliximab treatment in a patient with active Crohn disease and pyoderma gangrenosum. *Scand J Gastroenterol*. 2002;**37**:863-5.

20. Orchard TR, Wordsworth BP, Jewell DP. Peripheral arthropathies in inflammatory bowel disease: their articular distribution and natural history. *Gut* 1998;**42**:387-91.

21. Steer S, Jones H, Hibbert J *et al*. Low back pain, sacroiliitis, and the relationship with HLA-B27 in Crohn's disease. *J Rheumatol*. 2003;**30**:518-22.

22. de Vlam K, Mielants H, Cuvelier C *et al*. Spondyloarthropathy is underestimated in inflammatory bowel disease: prevalence and HLA association. *J Rheumatol*. 2000;**27**:2860-5.

23. Orchard TR, Wordsworth BP, Jewell DP. Peripheral arthropathies in inflammatory bowel disease: their articular distribution and natural history. *Gut* 1998;**42**:387-91.

24. Purrmann J, Zeidler H, Bertrams J *et al*. HLA antigens in ankylosing spondylitis associated with Crohn's disease. Increased frequency of the HLA phenotype B27,B44. *J Rheumatol*. 1988;**15**:1658-61.

25. Palm O, Moum B, Jahnsen J *et al*. The prevalence and incidence of peripheral arthritis in patients with inflammatory bowel disease, a prospective population-based study (the IBSEN study). *Rheumatology*. *(Oxford)* 2001;**40**:1256-61.

26. Orchard TR, Dhar A, Simmons JD *et al*. MHC class I chain-like gene A (MICA) and its associations with inflammatory bowel disease and peripheral arthropathy. *Clin Exp Immunol*. 2001;**126**:437-40.

27. Mattila J, Aitola P, Matikainen M. Liver lesions found at colectomy in ulcerative colitis: correlation between histological findings and biochemical parameters. *J Clin Pathol*. 1994;**47**:1019-21.

28. Perdigoto R, Carpenter HA, Czaja AJ. Frequency and significance of chronic ulcerative colitis in severe corticosteroid-treated autoimmune hepatitis. *J Hepatol*. 1992;**14**:325-31.

29. Broome U, Glaumann H, Hultcrantz R. Liver histology and follow up of 68 patients with ulcerative colitis and normal liver function tests. *Gut* 1990;**31**:468-72.

30. Lee YM, Kaplan MM. Primary sclerosing cholangitis. *N Engl J Med*. 1995;**332**:924-33.

31. Ludwig J, Barham SS, LaRusso NF *et al*. Morphologic features of chronic hepatitis associated with primary sclerosing cholangitis and chronic ulcerative colitis. *Hepatology* 1981;**1**: 632-40.

32. Chazouilleres O, Poupon R, Capron JP *et al*. Ursodeoxycholic acid for primary sclerosing cholangitis. *J Hepatol*. 1990;**11**:120-3.

33. Caprilli R, Viscido A, Guagnozzi D. Review article: biological agents in the treatment of Crohn's disease. *Aliment Pharmacol Ther*. 2002;**16**:1579-90.

34. Sutherland L, Roth D, Beck P *et al*. Oral 5-aminosalicylic acid for inducing remission in ulcerative colitis. [Review] [22 refs]. *Cochrane Database of Systematic Reviews [computer file]* 2000;CD000543.

35. Courtney MG, Nunes DP, Bergin CF *et al*. Randomised comparison of olsalazine and mesalazine in prevention of relapses in ulcerative colitis. *Lancet* 1992;**339**:1279-81.

36. Travis SP. Which 5-ASA? *Gut* 2002;*51*:548-9.

37. Eaden J, Abrams K, Ekbom A *et al*. Colorectal cancer prevention in ulcerative colitis: a case-control study. *Aliment Pharmacol Ther*. 2000;**14**:145-53.

38. Singleton JW, Hanauer SB, Gitnick GL *et al*. Mesalamine capsules for treatment of active Crohn's disease. *Gastroenterology* 1993;**104**:1301.

39. Hawthorne AB, Hawkey CJ. Immunosuppressive drugs in inflammatory bowel disease. A review of their mechanisms of efficacy and place in therapy. *Drugs* 1989;**38**:267-88.

40. Summers RW, Switz DM, Sessions JT jr *et al*. National Cooperative Crohn's disease Study: Results of drug treatment. *Gastroenterology* 1979;**77**:847-69.

41. Malchow H, Ewe K, Brandes JW *et al*. European Cooperative Crohn's Disease Study (ECCDS): results of drug treatment. *Gastroenterology* 1984;**86**:249-66.

42. Modigliani R, Mary JY, Simon JF *et al*. Clinical, biological, and endoscopic picture of attacks of Crohn's disease. Evolution on prednisolone. Groupe d'Etude Therapeutique des Affections Inflammatoires Digestives. *Gastroenterology* 1990;**98**:811-8.

43. Truelove SC, Watkinson G, Draper G. Comparison of corticosteroid and sulphasalazine therapy in ulcerative colitis. *Br Med J*. 1962;**5321**:1708-11.

44. Lennard-Jones, Longmore AJ, Newell AC. An assessment of prednisone, salazopyrine, and topical hydrocortisone hemisuccinate used as out-patient treatment for ulcerative colitis. *Gut* 1960;**1**:217-22.

45. Baron JH, Connell AM, Kanaghinis TG *et al*. Out-patient treatment of ulcerative colitis. Comparison between three doses of oral prednisone. *Br Med J*. 1962;**5302**:441-3.

46. Lang KA, Peppercorn MA. Promising new agents for the treatment of inflammatory bowel disorders. *Drugs R D*. 1999;**1**:237-44.

47. Mulder CJ, Tytgat GN. Review article: topical corticosteroids in inflammatory bowel disease. *Aliment Pharmacol Ther*. 1993;**7**:125-30.

48. Hanauer SB, Robinson M, Pruitt R *et al*. Budesonide enema for the treatment of active, distal ulcerative colitis and proctitis: a dose-ranging study. U.S. Budesonide enema study group. *Gastroenterology* 1998;**115**:525-32.

49. Marshall JK, Irvine EJ. Rectal corticosteroids versus alternative treatments in ulcerative colitis: A meta-analysis. *Gut* 1997;**40**:775-81.

50. Hanauer SB. Dose-ranging study of mesalamine (PENTASA) enemas in the treatment of acute ulcerative proctosigmoiditis: results of a multicentered placebo-controlled trial. The U.S. PENTASA Enema Study Group. *Inflamm Bowel Dis*. 1998;**4**:79-83.

51. Gionchetti P, Rizzello F, Venturi A *et al*. Comparison of mesalazine suppositories in proctitis and distal proctosigmoiditis. *Aliment Pharmacol Ther*. 1997;**11**:1053-7.

52. Marteau P, Crand J, Foucault M *et al*. Use of mesalazine slow release suppositories 1 g three times per week to maintain remission of ulcerative proctitis: a randomised double blind placebo controlled multicentre study. *Gut* 1998;**42**:195-9.

53. Sutherland L, Singleton J, Sessions J *et al*. Double blind, placebo controlled trial of metronidazole in Crohn's disease. *Gut* 1991;**32**:1071-5.

54. Colombel JF, Lemann M, Cassagnou M *et al*. A controlled trial comparing ciprofloxacin with mesalazine for the treatment of active Crohn's disease. Groupe d'Etudes Therapeutiques des Affections Inflammatoires Digestives (GETAID). *Am J Gastroenterol*. 1999;**94**:674-8.

55. Borgaonkar MR, MacIntosh DG, Fardy JM. A meta-analysis of antimycobacterial therapy for Crohn's disease. *Am J Gastroenterol*. 2000;**95**:725-9.

56. Sandborn W, Sutherland L, Pearson D *et al*. Azathioprine or 6-mercaptopurine for inducing remission of Crohn's disease. *Cochrane Database Syst Rev*. 2000;CD000545.

57. Pearson DC, May GR, Fick G *et al*. Azathioprine for maintaining remission of Crohn's disease. *Cochrane Database Syst Rev*. 2000;CD000067.

58. McGovern DP, Travis SP, Duley J *et al*. Azathioprine intolerance in patients with IBD may be imidazole-related and is independent of TPMT activity. *Gastroenterology* 2002;**122**:838-9.

59. Lennard L, Gibson BE, Nicole T *et al*. Congenital thiopurine methyltransferase deficiency and 6-mercaptopurine toxicity during treatment for acute lymphoblastic leukaemia. *Arch Dis Child* 1993;**69**:577-9.

60. Colombel J-F, Ferrari N, Debuysere H *et al*. Genotypic analysis of Thiopurine S-Methyltransferase in patients with Crohn's disease and severe myelopsuppression during Azathioprine therapy. *Gastroenterology* 2000;**118**:1025-30.

61. Campbell S, Kingstone K, Ghosh S. Relevance of thiopurine methyltransferase activity in inflammatory bowel disease patients maintained on low-dose azathioprine. *Aliment Pharmacol Ther* 2002;**16**:389-98.

62. Fraser AG, Orchard TR, Jewell DP. The efficacy of azathioprine for the treatment of inflammatory bowel disease: a 30 year review. *Gut* 2002;50:485-9.

63. Francella A, Dyan A, Bodian C *et al*. The safety of 6-mercaptopurine for childbearing patients with inflammatory bowel disease: a retrospective cohort study. *Gastroenterology* 2003;**124**:9-17.

64. Connell WR, Kamm MA, Ritchie JK *et al*. Bone marrow toxicity caused by azathioprine in inflammatory bowel disease: 27 years of experience. *Gut* 1993;**34**:1081-5.

65. Lewis JD, Bilker WB, Brensinger C *et al*. Inflammatory bowel disease is not associated with an increased risk of lymphoma. *Gastroenterology* 2001;**121**:1080-7.

66. Lewis JD, Schwartz JS, Lichtenstein GR. Azathioprine for maintenance of remission in Crohn's disease: benefits outweigh the risk of lymphoma. *Gastroenterology* 2000;**118**:1018-24.

67. Feagan BG, Rochon J, Fedorak RN *et al*. Methotrexate for the treatment of Crohn's disease. The North American Crohn's Study Group Investigators. *N Engl J .Med*. 1995;**332**:292-7.

68. Feagan BG, Fedorak RN, Irvine EJ *et al*. A comparison of methotrexate with placebo for the maintenance of remission in Crohn's disease. North American Crohn's Study Group Investigators. *N Engl J Med*. 2000;**342**:1627-32.

69. Kozarek RA, Patterson DJ, Gelfand MD *et al*. Methotrexate induces clinical and histologic remission in patients with refractory inflammatory bowel disease. *Ann Intern Med*. 1989;**110**:353-6.

70. Oren R, Arber N, Odes S *et al*. Methotrexate in chronic active ulcerative colitis: a double-blind, randomized, Israeli multicenter trial. *Gastroenterology* 1996;**110**:1416-21.

71. Fraser AG, Morton D, McGovern D *et al*. The efficacy of methotrexate for maintaining remission in inflammatory bowel disease. *Aliment Pharmacol Ther*. 2002;**16**:693-7.

72. Hamilton RA, Kremer JM. Why intramuscular methotrexate may be more efficacious than oral dosing in patients with rheumatoid arthritis. *Br J Rheumatol*. 1997;**36**:86-90.

73. Te HS, Schiano TD, Kuan SF *et al*. Hepatic effects of long-term methotrexate use in the treatment of inflammatory bowel disease. *Am J Gastroenterol*. 2000;**95**:3150-6.

74. Kremer JM, Alarcon GS, Weinblatt ME *et al*. Clinical, laboratory, radiographic, and histopathologic features of methotrexate-associated lung injury in patients with rheumatoid arthritis: a multicenter study with literature review. *Arthritis Rheum*. 1997;**40**:1829-37.

75. Baker K, Jewell DP. Cyclosporin for the treatment of severe inflammatory bowel disease. *Aliment Pharmacol Ther* 1989;**3**: 143-9.

76. Van Assche G, D'Haens G, Noman M *et al*. Randomized, double-blind comparison of 4 mg/kg versus 2 mg/kg intravenous cyclosporine in severe ulcerative colitis. *Gastroenterology* 2003;**125**:1025-31.

77. Actis GC, Aimo G, Priolo G, *et al*. Efficacy and efficiency of oral microemulsion cyclosporin versus intravenous and soft gelatin capsule cyclosporin in the treatment of severe steroid-refractory ulcerative colitis: an open-label retrospective trial. *Inflamm Bowel Dis*. 1998;**4**:276-9.

78. D'Haens G, Lemmens L, Geboes K *et al*. Intravenous cyclosporine versus intravenous corticosteroids as single therapy for severe attacks of ulcerative colitis. *Gastroenterology* 2001;**120**:1541-3.

79. Actis GC, Bresso F, Astegiano M *et al*. Safety and efficacy of azathioprine in the maintenance of ciclosporin-induced remission of ulcerative colitis. *Aliment Pharmacol Ther*. 2001;**15**:1307-11.

80. Feagan BG. Cyclosporin has no proven role as a therapy for Crohn's disease. *Inflamm Bowel Dis*. 1995;**1**:335-9.

81. Hawthorne AB. Ciclosporin and refractory colitis. *Eur J Gastroenterol Hepatol*. 2003;**15**:239-44.

82. Lichtiger S, Present DH, Kornbluth A *et al*. Cyclosporin in severe ulcerative colitis refractory to steroid therapy. *N Engl J Med*. 1994;**330**:1841-5.

83. Kornbluth A, Lichtiger S, Present DH. Long-term results of oral cyclosporin in patients with severe ulcerative colitis: A double-blind, randomized, multi-center trial. *Gastroenterology* 1994;**106**:A714.

84. Cohen RD, Stein R, Hanauer SB. Intravenous cyclosporin in ulceratice colitis: A five year experience. *Am J Gastroenterol*. 1999;**94**:1587-92.

85. Fernandez-Banares F, Bertran X, Esteve-Comas M *et al*. Azathioprine is useful in maintaining long-term remission induced by intravenous cyclosporine in steroid-refractory severe ulcerative colitis. *Am J Gastroenterol*. 1996;**91**:2498-9.

86. Goh J,.O'Morain CA. Review article: nutrition and adult inflammatory bowel disease. *Aliment Pharmacol Ther*. 2003;**17**:307-20.

87. Zachos M, Tondeur M, Griffiths AM. Enteral nutritional therapy for inducing remission of Crohn's disease. *Cochrane Database Syst Rev*. 2001;CD000542.

88. Griffiths AM. Enteral nutrition: the neglected primary therapy of active Crohn's disease. *J Pediatr Gastroenterol Nutr*. 2000;31:3-5.

89. Heuschkel RB,.Walker-Smith JA. Enteral nutrition in inflammatory bowel disease of childhood. JPEN *J Parenter Enteral Nutr*. 1999;**23**:S29-S32.

90. Graham TO, Kandil HM. Nutritional factors in inflammatory bowel disease. *Gastroenterol Clin North Am*. 2002;**31**:203-18.

91. Targan SR, Hanauer SB, van Deventer SJ *et al*. A short-term study of chimeric monoclonal antibody cA2 to tumor necrosis factor alpha for Crohn's disease. Crohn's Disease cA2 Study Group. *N Engl J Med*. 1997;**337**:1029-35.

92. Hanauer SB, Feagan BG, Lichtenstein GR *et al*. Maintenance infliximab for Crohn's disease: the ACCENT I randomised trial. *Lancet* 2002;**359**:1541-9.

93. Present DH, Rutgeerts P, Targan S *et al*. Infliximab for the treatment of fistulas in patients with Crohn's disease. *N Engl J Med*. 1999;**340**:1398-405.

94. Sands BE, Anderson FH, Bernstein CN *et al*. Infliximab maintenance therapy for fistulizing Crohn's disease. *N Engl J Med*. 2004;**350**:876-85.

95. Keane J, Gershon S, Wise RP *et al*. Tuberculosis associated with infliximab, a tumor necrosis factor alpha-neutralizing agent. *N Engl J Med*. 2001;**345**:1098-104.

96. Dunckley P, Jewell D. Management of acute severe colitis. *Best Pract Res Clin Gastroenterol*. 2003;**17**:89-103.

97. Leong AP, Londono-Schimmer EE, Phillips RK. Life-table analysis of stomal complications following ileostomy. *Br J Surg* 1994;**81**:727-9.

98. Fazio VW, Ziv Y, Church JM *et al*. Ileal pouch-anal anastomoses complications and function in 1005 patients. *Ann Surg*. 1995;**222**:120-7.

99. Andrews HA, Keighley MR, Alexander-Williams J *et al.* Strategy for management of distal ileal Crohn's disease. *Br J .Surg* 1991;**78**:679-82.

100. Fazio VW, Marchetti F, Church M *et al.* Effect of resection margins on the recurrence of Crohn's disease in the small bowel. A randomized controlled trial. *Ann Surg.* 1996;**224**:563-71.

101. Stebbing JF, Jewell DP, Kettlewell MG *et al.* Recurrence and reoperation after strictureplasty for obstructive Crohn's disease: long-term results [corrected]. *Br J Surg.* 1995;**82**:1471-4.

102. Yamamoto T, Bain IM, Mylonakis E, *et al.* Stapled functional end-to-end anastomosis versus sutured end-to-end anastomosis after ileocolonic resection in Crohn disease. *Scand J Gastroenterol.* 1999;**34**:708-13.

103. Edwards CM, George BD, Jewell DP *et al.* Role of a defunctioning stoma in the management of large bowel Crohn's disease. *Br J Surg* 2000;**87**:1063-6.

104. Yamamoto T, Keighley MR. Smoking and disease recurrence after operation for Crohn's disease. *Br J Surg* 2000;**87**:398-404.

105. Lochs H, Mayer M, Fleig WE *et al.* Prophylaxis of postoperative relapse in Crohn's disease with mesalamine: European Cooperative Crohn's Disease Study VI. *Gastroenterology* 2000;**118**:264-73.

106. Cottone M, Camma C. Mesalamine and relapse prevention in Crohn's disease. *Gastroenterology* 2000;**119:**597.

107. Korelitz BI, Hanauer S, Rutgeerts P, *et al.* Post-operative prophylaxis with 6-MP, 5-ASA or placebo in Crohn's disease: a 2 year multicenter trial. *Gastroenterology* 1998;**114**:A1011.

108. Travis S. Azathioprine for prevention of postoperative recurrence in Crohn's disease. *Eur J Gastroenterol Hepatol.* 2001;**13**:1277-9.

109. Sandborn W, McLeod R, Jewell D. Pharmacotherapy for inducing and maintaining remission in pouchitis. *Cochrane Database Syst Rev.* 2000;CD001176.

110. Gionchetti P, Rizzello F, Venturi A *et al.* Oral bacteriotherapy as maintenance treatment in patients with chronic pouchitis: a double-blind, placebo-controlled trial. *Gastroenterology* 2000;**119**:305-9.

111. Jawhari A, Kamm MA, Ong C *et al*. Intra-abdominal and pelvic abscess in Crohn's disease: results of noninvasive and surgical management. *Br J Surg*. 1998;**85**:367-71.

112. Schwartz DA, Pemberton JH, Sandborn WJ. Diagnosis and treatment of perianal fistulas in Crohn disease. *Ann Intern Med*. 2001;**135**:906-18.

113. Loftus EV, Jr., Crowson CS, Sandborn WJ *et al*. Long-term fracture risk in patients with Crohn's disease: a population-based study in Olmsted County, Minnesota. *Gastroenterology* 2002;**123**:468-75.

114. Stockbrugger RW, Schoon EJ, Bollani S *et al*. Discordance between the degree of osteopenia and the prevalence of spontaneous vertebral fractures in Crohn's disease. *Aliment Pharmacol Ther*. 2002;**16**:1519-27.

115. van Staa TP, Cooper C, Brusse LS *et al*. Inflammatory bowel disease and the risk of fracture. *Gastroenterology* 2003;**125**: 1591-7.

116. Robinson RJ, Krzywicki T, Almond L *et al*. Effect of a low-impact exercise program on bone mineral density in Crohn's disease: a randomized controlled trial. *Gastroenterology* 1998;**115**:36-41.

117. Haderslev KV, Tjellesen L, Sorensen HA *et al*. Alendronate increases lumbar spine bone mineral density in patients with Crohn's disease. *Gastroenterology* 2000;**119**:639-46.

118. Clements D, Compston JE, Evans WD *et al*. Hormone replacement therapy prevents bone loss in patients with inflammatory bowel disease. *Gut* 1993;**34**:1543-6.

119. Eaden JA, Abrams KR, Mayberry JF. The risk of colorectal cancer in ulcerative colitis: a meta-analysis. *Gut* 2001;**48**:526-35.

120. Langholz E, Munkholm P, Davidsen M *et al*. Colorectal cancer risk and mortality in patients with ulcerative colitis. *Gastroenterology* 1992;**103**:1444-51.

121. Gillen CD, Andrews HA, Prior P *et al*. Crohn's disease and colorectal cancer. *Gut* 1994;**35**:651-5.

122. Ekbom A, Helmick C, Zack M *et al*. Ulcerative colitis and colorectal cancer. A population-based study. *N Engl J Med*. 1990;**323**:1228-33.

123. Lennard-Jones JE, Melville DM, Morson BC *et al*. Precancer and cancer in extensive ulcerative colitis: findings among 401 patients over 22 years. *Gut* 1990;**31**:800-6.

124. Soetikno RM, Lin OS, Heidenreich PA *et al*. Increased risk of colorectal neoplasia in patients with primary sclerosing cholangitis and ulcerative colitis: a meta-analysis. *Gastrointest Endosc*. 2002;**56**:48-54.

125. Gasche C. Anemia in IBD: the overlooked villain. *Inflamm Bowel Dis*. 2000;**6**:142-50.

126. Thomson AB, Brust R, Ali MA *et al*. Iron deficiency in inflammatory bowel disease. Diagnostic efficacy of serum ferritin. *Am J Dig Dis*. 1978;**23**:705-9.

127. Gasche C, Waldhoer T, Feichtenschlager T *et al*. Prediction of response to iron sucrose in inflammatory bowel disease-associated anemia. *Am J Gastroenterol*. 2001;**96**:2382-7.

128. Demirturk L, Hulagu S, Yaylaci M *et al*. Serum erythropoietin levels in patients with severe anemia secondary to inflammatory bowel disease and the use of recombinant human erythropoietin in patients with anemia refractory to treatment. *Dis Colon Rectum*. 1995;**38**:896-7.

129. Eaden JA, Mayberry JF. Guidelines for screening and surveillance of asymptomatic colorectal cancer in patients with inflammatory bowel disease. *Gut* 2002;**51 Suppl 5**:V10-V12.

130. Connell WR, Talbot IC, Harpaz N *et al*. Clinicopathological characteristics of colorectal carcinoma complicating ulcerative colitis. *Gut* 1994;**35**:1419-23.

131. Axon AT. Cancer surveillance in ulcerative colitis—a time for reappraisal. *Gut* 1994;**35**:587-9.

132. Moody GA, Probert C, Jayanthi V *et al*. The effects of chronic ill health and treatment with sulphasalazine on fertility amongst men and women with inflammatory bowel disease in Leicestershire. *Int J Colorectal Dis*. 1997;**12**:220-4.

133. O'Morain C, Smethurst P, Dore CJ, Levi AJ. Reversible male infertility due to sulphasalazine: studies in man and rat. *Gut* 1984;**25**:1078-84.

134. Dejaco C, Mittermaier C, Reinisch W *et al*. Azathioprine treatment and male fertility in inflammatory bowel disease. *Gastroenterology* 2001;**121**:1048-53.

135. Rajapakse RO, Korelitz BI, Zlatanic J *et al*. Outcome of pregnancies when fathers are treated with 6-mercaptopurine for inflammatory bowel disease. *Am J Gastroenterol*. 2000;**95**:684-8.

136. Alstead EM, Nelson-Piercy C. Inflammatory bowel disease in pregnancy. *Gut* 2003;**52**:159-61.

137. Olsen KO, Joelsson M, Laurberg S *et al*. Fertility after ileal pouch-anal anastomosis in women with ulcerative colitis. *Br J Surg* 1999;**86**:493-5.

138. Korelitz BI. Inflammatory bowel disease and pregnancy. Gastroenterol. *Clin North Am*. 1998;**27**:213-24.

139. Kornfeld D, Cnattingius S, Ekbom A. Pregnancy outcomes in women with inflammatory bowel disease—a population-based cohort study. *Am J Obstet Gynecol*. 1997;**177**:942-6.

140. Norgard B, Fonager K, Sorensen HT *et al*. Birth outcomes of women with ulcerative colitis: a nationwide Danish cohort study. *Am J Gastroenterol*. 2000;**95**:3165-70.

141. Fonager K, Sorensen HT, Olsen J *et al*. Pregnancy outcome for women with Crohn's disease: a follow-up study based on linkage between national registries. *Am J Gastroenterol*. 1998;**93**:2426-30.

142. Diav-Citrin O, Park YH, Veerasuntharam G *et al*. The safety of mesalamine in human pregnancy: a prospective controlled cohort study. *Gastroenterology* 1998;**114**:23-8.

143. Koren G, Pastuszak A, Ito S. Drugs in pregnancy. *N Engl J Med*. 1998;**338**:1128-37.

144. Ferrero S, Ragni N. Inflammatory bowel disease: management issues during pregnancy. *Arch Gynecol Obstet*. 2003.

145. Katz JA, Lichtenstein GR, Keenan GF, *et al*. Outcome of pregnancy in women receiving Remicade (infliximab) for the treatment of Crohn's disease and rheumatoid arthritis. *Gastroenterology* 2001;**120**:A366.

146. Ost L, Wettrell G, Bjorkhem I *et al*. Prednisolone excretion in human milk. *J Pediatr*. 1985;**106**:1008-11.

147. Polito JM, Childs B, Mellits ED *et al*. Crohn's disease: influence of age at diagnosis on site and clinical type of disease. *Gastroenterology* 1996;**111**:580-6.

148. Hyams JS, Davis P, Grancher K *et al*. Clinical outcome of ulcerative colitis in children. *J Pediatr*. 1996;**129**:81-8.

149. Cameron DJ. Upper and lower gastrointestinal endoscopy in children and adolescents with Crohn's disease: a prospective study. *J Gastroenterol Hepatol*. 1991;**6**:355-8.

150. Griffiths AM, Nguyen P, Smith C *et al*. Growth and clinical course of children with Crohn's disease. *Gut* 1993;**34**:939-43.

151. Motil KJ, Grand RJ, Davis-Kraft L *et al*. Growth failure in children with inflammatory bowel disease: a prospective study. *Gastroenterology* 1993;**105**:681-91.

152. Ruemmele FM, Roy CC, Levy E *et al*. Nutrition as primary therapy in pediatric Crohn's disease: fact or fantasy? *J Pediatr*. 2000;**136**:285-91.

153. Markowitz J, Grancher K, Kohn N *et al*. A multicenter trial of 6-mercaptopurine and prednisone in children with newly diagnosed Crohn's disease. *Gastroenterology* 2000;**119**:895-902.

154. Fuentes D, Torrente F, Keady S *et al*. High-dose azathioprine in children with inflammatory bowel disease. *Aliment Pharmacol Ther*. 2003;**17**:913-21.

155. Peeters M, Nevens H, Baert F *et al*. Familial aggregation in Crohn's disease: increased age-adjusted risk and concordance in clinical characteristics. *Gastroenterology* 1996;**111**:597-603.

156. Orholm M, Fonager K, Sorensen HT. Risk of ulcerative colitis and Crohn's disease among offspring of patients with chronic inflammatory bowel disease. *Am J Gastroenterol*. 1999;**94**:3236-8.

157. Bennett RA, Rubin PH, Present DH. Frequency of inflammatory bowel disease in offspring of couples both presenting with inflammatory bowel disease. *Gastroenterology* 1991;**100**:1638-43.

158. Winther KV, Jess T, Langholz E *et al*. Survival and cause-specific mortality in ulcerative colitis: follow-up of a population-based cohort in Copenhagen County. *Gastroenterology* 2003;**125**:1576-82.

159. Card T, Hubbard R, Logan RF. Mortality in inflammatory bowel disease: a population-based cohort study. *Gastroenterology* 2003;**125**:1583-90.

160. Carter M, Lobo A, Travis SPL. British Society of Gastroenterology guidelines for the management of inflammatory bowel disease in adults. *Gut* 2004 (in press).

Appendix 1 – Drugs

Drug	Trade name	Format	Preparation	Strengths	Dose	Comments	Precautions/side effects
Aminosalicylates							
						The main role for **oral 5-ASA** is maintenance of remission in ulcerative colitis. Individual 5-ASA derivatives all show comparable efficacy to sulfasalazine, but in a meta-analysis sulfasalazine had a modest therapeutic advantage for maintaining remission (odds ratio 1.29; confidence interval 1.08–1.57). [Sutherland LR, Roth DE, Beck PL. Alternatives to sulfasalazine: a meta-analysis of 5-ASA in the treatment of ulcerative colitis. *Inflamm Bowel Dis* 1997;**3**:65–78]. Side effects between new 5-ASA do not differ significantly [Loftus EV, Kane SV, Bjorkman D. Systematic review: short term adverse effects of 5-aminosalicylic acid agents in the treatment of ulcerative colitis. *Aliment Pharmacol Ther* 2004;**19**:179–89]. The main role for **topical 5-ASA** is as an adjunct to treatment of active, distal ulcerative colitis or proctitis. Topical mesalazine is more effective than topical steroid for distal colitis, but may be less well tolerated. As a rule, patients tolerate suppositories better than foam and foam better than liquid enemas. Foam and liquid enemas frequently bypass the rectum, so suppositories are best for proctitis. The optimal dose of topical mesalazine is 1 g/day. [Cohen RD, Woseth DM, Thisted RA, Hanauer SB. A meta-analysis and overview of the literature on treatment options for left-sided ulcerative colitis and ulcerative proctitis. *Am J Gastroenterol* 2000;**95**:1263–1276].	
Balsalazide	Colazide®	Oral	Capsules	750 mg	Acute dose: 2.25 g three times/day; maintenance: 1.5 g twice/day; not recommended in children		Precautions: kidney disease, allergy to aspirin and aspirin-like products, pregnancy or breast-feeding. Side effects: headache, belly pain/cramps, nausea/vomiting, diarrhoea, muscle aches/pains, lung infections

Drug	Trade name	Format	Preparation	Strengths	Dose	Comments	Precautions/side effects
Aminosalicylates							
Mesalazine	Asacol® MR	Oral	Tablets	400 mg	Acute dose: 2.4 g/day in divided doses; maintenance dose: 1.2–2.4 g/day in divided doses; not recommended in children	Possibly less effective for distal disease. Should be prescribed by brand name.	Common side effects (≤ 10%): nausea, diarrhoea, abdominal pain, rash, headache (a systematic review has not shown significant differences between 5-ASA derivatives)
	Asacol®	Topical	Suppositories	250 mg or 500 mg	500 mg twice/day; not recommended in children	Twice-daily dosing needed for adequate dose	Rare side effects (< 1%): pancreatitis, interstitial nephritis (may be more common than with sulfasalazine), hepatitis, leucopenia, thrombocytopenia, aplastic anaemia, myocarditis, fibrosing alveolitis, systemic lupus erythematosus-like syndrome
			Foam enema	1g/metered application	Acute dose: 1 g at night (rectosigmoid region affected); 2 g at night (descending colon affected); not recommended in children	Useful for refractory distal ulcerative colitis	

Drug	Trade name	Format	Preparation	Strengths	Dose	Comments	Precautions/side effects
Aminosalicylates							
Mesalazine	Ipocol®	Oral	Tablets	400 mg	Acute dose: 2.4 g/day in divided doses; maintenance dose: 1.2–2.4 g/day in divided doses; not recommended in children	Generic mesalazine; no controlled trials. Cannot be considered interchangeable with Asacol	Common side effects (≤ 10%): nausea, diarrhoea, abdominal pain, rash, headache (a systematic review has not shown significant differences between 5-ASA derivatives) Rare side effects (< 1%): pancreatitis, interstitial nephritis (may be more common than with sulfasalazine), hepatitis, leucopenia, thrombocytopenia, aplastic anaemia, myocarditis, fibrosing alveolitis, systemic lupus erythematosus-like syndrome
	Mesren®	Oral	Tablets	400 mg	Acute dose: 2.4 g in divided doses; not recommended in children	Generic mesalazine; no controlled trials. Release of mesalazine may be prevented by preparations that lower stool pH (e.g. lactulose)	
	Salofalk®	Oral	Tablets	250 mg	500 mg–1 g; three times/day; not recommended in children		

Drug	Trade name	Format	Preparation	Strengths	Dose	Comments	Precautions/side effects
Aminosalicylates							
Mesalazine	Salofalk®	Oral	Granules	500 mg/sachet	Acute dose: 500 mg–1 g three times/day; maintenance dose: 500 mg three times/day; in child > 6 years: half dose if BW < 40 kg, full dose if BW > 40 kg		Common side effects (≤ 10%): nausea, diarrhoea, abdominal pain, rash, headache (a systematic review has not shown significant differences between 5-ASA derivatives) Rare side effects (< 1%): pancreatitis, interstitial nephritis (may be more common than with sulfasalazine), hepatitis, leucopenia, thrombocytopenia, aplastic anaemia, myocarditis, fibrosing alveolitis, systemic lupus erythematosus-like syndrome
		Topical	Suppositories	500 mg	500 mg–1 g two to three times/day; not recommended in children	Twice-daily dosing needed for adequate dose	
			Liquid enema	2 g/59-ml pack	2 g once/day; not recommended in children	Dose unnecessarily high	
			Rectal foam	1g/metered application	2 g at bedtime; not recommended in children		

Drug	Trade name	Format	Preparation	Strengths	Dose	Comments	Precautions/side effects
Aminosalicylates							
Mesalazine	Pentasa®	Oral	Slow-release tablets	500 mg	Acute dose: up to 4 g/day in 2–3 divided doses; maintenance dose: 1.5 g/day in 2–3 divided doses; not recommended in child < 15 years	Useful for Crohn's disease as well as ulcerative colitis	Common side effects (≤ 10%): nausea, diarrhoea, abdominal pain, rash, headache (a systematic review has not shown significant differences between 5-ASA derivatives) Rare side effects (< 1%): pancreatitis, interstitial nephritis (may be more common than with sulfasalazine), hepatitis, leucopenia, thrombocytopenia, aplastic anaemia, myocarditis, fibrosing alveolitis, systemic lupus erythematosus-like syndrome
			Prolonged release granules	1 g/sachet	Acute dose: up to 4 g/day in 2–4 divided doses; maintenance dose: 2 g/day in two divided doses; not recommended in child < 12 years		
		Topical	Liquid enema	1 g/100-ml pack	1 g at bedtime; not recommended in children		
			Suppositories	1 g	Acute/maintenance dose: 1 g/day; not recommended in child < 15 years	Best suppository for acute proctitis	

Drug	Trade name	Format	Preparation	Strengths	Dose	Comments	Precautions/side effects
Aminosalicylates							
Olsalazine	Dipentum®	Oral	Capsules	250 mg	Acute dose: 1–3 g/day in 2–3 divided doses; maintenance dose: 500 mg twice/day; not recommended in children	Useful maintenance therapy in distal disease/ proctitis	Precautions: pregnancy, breast-feeding, kidney disease, blood disorders, allergy to aspirin/ aspirin-like products Side effects: rash, abdominal cramps, nausea, dyspepsia, anaemia, arthralgia, neutropenia, thrombocytopenia, headache, diarrhoea
			Tablets	500 mg	Acute dose: 1–3 g/day in 2–3 divided doses; maintenance dose: 500 mg twice/day; not recommended in children		

Drug	Trade name	Format	Preparation	Strengths	Dose	Comments	Precautions/side effects
Aminosalicylates							
Sulfasalazine	Non-proprietary	Oral	Tablets	500 mg	Acute dose: 1–2 g four times/day (40–60 mg/kg/day in child > 2 years); maintenance dose: 500 mg four times/day (20–30 mg/kg/day in child > 2 years)		Common side effects (≤ 10%): nausea, vomiting, dyspepsia, headache, fever, rashes, reversible oligospermia Rare side effects (< 1%): neutropenia (much less common than for rheumatoid arthritis), folate deficiency, aplastic anaemia, pancreatitis, hepatitis, fibrosing alveolitis, Stevens-Johnson nephrotic syndrome, neurotoxicity, photosensitization
	Salazopyrin (EN-Tabs)®	Oral	Tablets	500 mg	Acute dose: 1–2 g four times/ day (40–60 mg/kg/day in child > 2 years); maintenance dose: 500 mg four times/day (20–30 mg/kg/day in child > 2 years)	Best for maintenance if tolerated	

Drug	Trade name	Format	Preparation	Strengths	Dose	Comments	Precautions/side effects
Aminosalicylates							
Sulfasalazine	Salazopyrin®	Oral	Suspension	250 mg/5 ml	Acute dose: 1–2 g four times/ day (40–60 mg/kg/day in child > 2 years); maintenance dose: 500 mg four times/day (20–30 mg/kg/day in child > 2 years)		Common side effects (≤ 10%): nausea, vomiting, dyspepsia, headache, fever, rashes, reversible oligospermia Rare side effects (< 1%): neutropenia (much less common than for rheumatoid arthritis), folate deficiency, aplastic anaemia, pancreatitis, hepatitis, fibrosing alveolitis, Stevens–Johnson nephrotic syndrome, neurotoxicity, photosensitization
		Topical	Suppositories	500 mg	500 mg–1 g twice/day; not recommended in children	Largely superseded by mesalazine suppositories	
			Liquid enema	3 g in 100-ml single-dose packs	3 g at night; not recommended in children	Almost no role	

Drug	Trade name	Format	Preparation	Strengths	Dose	Comments	Precautions/side effects
Corticosteroids							
Steroids are indicated for active ulcerative colitis or Crohn's disease; decisive treatment with full dose, reduced over 6–8 weeks is more effective than modest doses. Rapid dose reduction may lead to early relapse, but there is no place for steroids of any formulation in the maintenance of remission, since they are ineffective. Early introduction of an immunomodulator (azathioprine, etc.) is appropriate for patients who appear steroid-dependent.							
Budesonide	Budenofalk®	Oral	Capsules	3 mg	9 mg/day for 6 weeks, then 6 mg/day for 4 weeks; not recommended in children	Ileo-ascending Crohn's, but may be effective in Crohn's colitis. No place for maintenance.	Contraindications: diabetes, hypertension, osteoporosis, peptic ulcer disease, concurrent infection Short-term side effects: hyperglycaemia/hypokalaemia, mood changes/psychosis/ disturbed sleep, masking/ induction of intestinal perforation/infection, avascular osteonecrosis, reactivation of tuberculosis/chickenpox, weight gain/fluid retention/acne, peptic ulcer
	Entocort®	Oral	CR capsules	3 mg	9 mg/day for 6 weeks, then 6 mg/day for 4 weeks; not recommended in children	Ileo-ascending Crohn's. No place for maintenance.	
		Topical	Liquid enema	2 mg/ 100-ml enema	2 mg at bedtime for 4 weeks; not recommended in children	Generally less well tolerated than foam enema	Long-term side effects: purpura/moon facies/ hirsutism/proximal myopathy, adrenocortical suppression, osteoporosis, growth retardation, hypertension, cataract/glaucoma, skin-thinning

Drug	Trade name	Format	Preparation	Strengths	Dose	Comments	Precautions/side effects
Corticosteroids							
Hydro-cortisone	Colifoam®	Topical	Foam enema	Hydrocortisone acetate 10%	125 mg once or twice/day; not usually recommended in children	Cheaper but less effective than 5-ASA enemas	Contraindications: diabetes, hypertension, osteoporosis, peptic ulcer disease, concurrent infection
	Efcortesol®	iv injection	1-ml ampoule	100 mg/ml	400 mg/day (25 mg in child ≤1 year: 50 mg in child 1–5 years; 100 mg in child 6–12 years)	For severe ulcerative colitis or Crohn's disease in hospitalized patients	Short-term side effects: hyperglycaemia/hypokalaemia. mood changes/psychosis/ disturbed sleep, masking/ induction of intestinal perforation/infection, avascular osteonecrosis, reactivation of tuberculosis/chickenpox, weight gain/fluid retention/acne, peptic ulcer
	Solu-Cortef®	iv injection	Powder for reconstitution	100 mg/vial			
Prednisolone	Non-proprietary	Oral	Tablets	1/5/25 mg; 2.5/5 mg (e/c)	20–40 mg/day in single or divided doses until remission, then reduced doses. 1–1.5mg/kg/day in children, guided by paediatric specialist	Active Crohn's or ulcerative colitis. No place for maintenance.	Long-term side effects: purpura/moon facies/ hirsutism/proximal myopathy, adrenocortical suppression, osteoporosis, growth retardation, hypertension, cataract/glaucoma, skin-thinning

Drug	Trade name	Format	Preparation	Strengths	Dose	Comments	Precautions/side effects
Corticosteroids							
Prednisolone	Non-proprietary	Oral	Soluble tablets	5 mg	20–40 mg/day in single or divided doses until remission, then reduced doses 1–1.5mg/kg/day in children, guided by paediatric specialist	As above	Contraindications: diabetes, hypertension, osteoporosis, peptic ulcer disease, concurrent infection Short-term side effects: hyperglycaemia/hypokalaemia, mood changes/psychosis/ disturbed sleep, masking/ induction of intestinal perforation/infection, avascular osteonecrosis, reactivation of tuberculosis/chickenpox, weight gain/fluid retention/acne, peptic ulcer Long-term side effects: purpura/moon facies/ hirsutism/proximal myopathy, adrenocortical suppression, osteoporosis, growth retardation, hypertension, cataract/glaucoma, skin-thinning
	Predenema®	Topical	Liquid enema	20 mg/ 100-ml single-dose disposable pack	20 mg at bedtime; not recommended in children	Generally less well tolerated than foam	
	Predfoam®	Topical	Foam enema	20 mg/ metered application	20 mg at bedtime for 2–4 weeks; not recommended in children	Cheaper, but less effective than 5-ASA enemas	

Drug	Trade name	Format	Preparation	Strengths	Dose	Comments	Precautions/side effects
Corticosteroids							
Prednisolone	Predsol®	Topical	Liquid enema	20 mg/ 100-ml single-dose disposable pack	20 mg at bedtime for 2–4 weeks; not recommended in children	Generally less well tolerated than foam	Contraindications: diabetes, hypertension, osteoporosis, peptic ulcer disease, concurrent infection
			Suppositories	5 mg	5 mg once to twice/day; not usually recomm-ended in children		Short-term side effects: hyperglycaemia/hypokalaemia, mood changes/psychosis/ disturbed sleep, masking/ induction of intestinal perforation/infection, avascular osteonecrosis, reactivation of tuberculosis/chickenpox, weight gain/fluid retention/acne, peptic ulcer
	Solu-Medrone®	iv injection	Powder for reconstitution	40 mg methylpre-dnisolone	60 mg/day; not usually recommended in children	For severe ulcerative colitis or Crohn's disease in hospitalized patients	Long-term side effects: purpura/moon facies/ hirsutism/proximal myopathy, adrenocortical suppression, osteoporosis, growth retardation, hypertension, cataract/glaucoma, skin-thinning

Azathioprine/mercaptopurine

The main role for azathioprine or mercaptopurine are as steroid-sparing agents for those patients with ulcerative colitis or Crohn's disease whose symptoms recur as the dose of prednisolone is tapered or recur soon after prednisolone is stopped: patients who require two or more corticosteroids courses within a calendar year; those whose disease relapses as the dose of steroid is reduced below 15 mg; or relapses within 6 weeks of stopping steroid steroids or postoperative prophylaxis of complex (fistulating or extensive) Crohn's disease. Neither azathioprine nor mercaptopurine is licensed in the UK for treatment of UC or CD, but both have been widely used for decades [Travis SPL, editor. Recent advances in immunomodulation in the treatment of inflammatory bowel disease: review in depth. *Eur J Gastroenterol Hepatol* 2003;**15**:215–248].

Drug	Trade name	Format	Preparation	Strengths	Dose	Comments	Precautions/side effects
Azathioprine	Non-proprietary	Oral	Tablets	25 mg	1.5–2.5 mg/kg/day (to be reduced in hepatic/renal impairment); same dose in children		Precautions: hepatic/renal impairment, breast-feeding Contraindications: previous hypersensitivity, pregnancy, concurrent allopurinol therapy
	Imuran®	Oral	Tablets	25 mg	1.5–2.5 mg/kg/day (to be reduced in hepatic/renal impairment); same dose in children		Allergy-type side effects: characteristically occur within 3–4 weeks in up to 25% of individuals; many who do not tolerate azathioprine may tolerate mercaptopurine: fever/ rigors/myalgia/arthralgia/malaise /nausea/vomiting, diarrhoea, jaundice (hepatitic or cholestatic pattern), pancreatitis /pneumonitis Dose-dependent side effects: bone-marrow suppression, hair loss, possible increased risk of lymphoma during long-term therapy
		iv injection	Powder for reconstitution	50-mg vial (as sodium salt)		No indication in UC or CD	
Mercapto-purine	Puri-Nethol®	Oral	Tablets	50 mg	0.75–1.25 mg/kg/ day (to be reduced in hepatic/renal impairment); same dose in children	Can be tolerated by up to 75% of patients with gastrointestinal intolerance to azathioprine	

Drug	Trade name	Format	Preparation	Strengths	Dose	Comments	Precautions/side effects
Ciclosporin							
Ciclosporin is only used for severe ulcerative colitis that does not respond to steroids, or when steroids are considered inappropriate. It is almost invariably initiated in hospital under specialist supervision, and used for about 3 months. Topical enemas can be specially made and are occasionally used for refractory distal colitis. [Travis SPL, editor. Recent advances in immunomodulation in the treatment of inflammatory bowel disease: review in depth. *Eur J Gastroenterol Hepatol* 2003;**15**:215–248].							
Ciclosporin	Neoral®	Oral	Capsules	10/25/50/ 100 mg	5 mg/kg/day; not usually recommended in children	Dose adjusted to maintain trough ciclosporin level at 150–300 ng/ml. Dose reduction with mild renal impairment (20–30% reduction in creatinine clearance).	Absolute contraindications: established renal impairment (> 20–30% reduction in baseline creatinine clearance), acute porphyria, hypocholesterolaemia (< 3.0 mmol/l)/ hypomagnesaemia (< 0.5 mmol/l), pregnancy Relative contraindications: previous malignancy/hypertension/epilepsy Side effects: dose-dependent increase in urea and creatinine (common, early and reversible) and nephrotoxicity (less common, late, chronic, irreversible), hypertension/ hyperkalaemia/hypertrichosis/ gingival hypertrophy, tremor/ headache/rash, hepatic dysfunction/ gastrointestinal disturbances/pancreatitis, neurotoxicity – convulsions/ paraesthesia/myopathy/ neuropathy/ confusion
	Sandimmun®	iv infusion	Concentrate for iv infusion	50 mg/ml (1 or 5-ml ampoule)	2 mg/kg/day infusion over 6 hr; not usually recommended in children	Dose adjusted to maintain ciclosporin level at 150–300 ng/ml	

Drug	Trade name	Format	Preparation	Strengths	Dose	Comments	Precautions/side effects

Methotrexate

Methotrexate is an effective treatment for inducing remission or preventing relapse in Crohn's disease. At present, the role of methotrexate is in the treatment of active or relapsing Crohn's disease for patients who are refractory to or intolerant of azathioprine or mecaptopurine. [Travis SPL, editor. Recent advances in immunomodulation in the treatment of inflammatory bowel disease: review in depth. *Eur J Gastroenterol Hepatol* 2003;**15**:215–248].

Drug	Trade name	Format	Preparation	Strengths	Dose	Comments	Precautions/side effects
Methotrexate	Non-proprietary	Oral	Tablets	2.5/10 mg	15–25mg once/week; not usually recommended in children	Administration on a *Monday* is easy to remember; concomitant folic acid 5 mg (on a *Friday*) to reduce intolerance	Contraindications: pregnancy (teratogenic and abortifacient), significant renal impairment, liver or lung disease, breast-feeding, immunodeficiency syndromes, acute porphyria Side effects (about 15% patients affected): bone-marrow suppression, nausea, vomiting, stomatitis, liver toxicity (fibrosis/cirrhosis) on prolonged (> 3 years) use, photosensitization/rash, pulmonary fibrosis/pneumonitis (rare)
		im injection	Concentrtate for im injections	2.5/25/100 mg/ml			

Antitumour necrosis factor α antibody

National guidelines govern the use of infliximab. In the UK, it is limited to patients with severe active Crohn's disease (Harvey-Bradshaw index > 8, Crohn's disease activity index > 300) refractory or intolerant to steroids and immunosuppression, for whom surgery is inappropriate. Although licensed for maintenance therapy in Crohn's disease, it is generally administered intermittently as need arises. [Travis SPL, editor. Recent advances in immunomodulation in the treatment of inflammatory bowel disease: review in depth. *Eur J Gastroenterol Hepatol* 2003;**15**:215–248].

Drug	Trade name	Format	Preparation	Strengths	Dose	Comments	Precautions/side effects
Infliximab	Remicade®	iv infusion	Powder for reconstitution	100 mg/vial	5 mg/kg as single iv infusion for refractory, active Crohn's disease; repeated doses of 5 mg/kg at 2 and 6 weeks for fistulating disease	Administered under specialist supervision according to NICE guidelines	Contraindications: abscess, infection, intestinal strictures, previous TB, cardiac failure, multiple sclerosis (rare), previous/current malignancy, ulcerative colitis (ineffective for moderate refractory disease), pregnancy/breast-feeding, hypersensitivity to previous infusion (pretreat with hydrocortisone 100–200 mg) Side effects: hypersensitivity reactions during infusion (~20%) but anaphylaxis exceptional, five-fold increase in risk of TB, chest pain/dyspnoea/nausea/rash/fever, headache/nausea/fatigue, immunogenicity (serum sickness and lupus-like syndrome reported), malignancy/lymphoma (theoretical risk), exacerbation of strictures and intestinal obstruction

Appendix 2 – Monitoring advice

Summary of monitoring advice for drugs used in inflammatory bowel disease

Sulfasalazine and aminosalicylates	*Committee on Safety of Medicines recommendation*: report unexplained bleeding, easy bruising, purpura, sore throat, fever or malaise for check full blood count.
Sulfasalazine	Full blood count and liver function tests monthly for 1st 3 months (*British National Formulary*). Thereafter, 3–12-monthly full blood count/full blood count/liver function tests/renal function. Evidence of practical value of monitoring is lacking.
Mesalazine/ 5-aminosalicylates	Prescribers should be alert to the possibility of interstitial nephritis, but evidence of practical value of monitoring of renal function is lacking.
Corticosteroids	Blood pressure/blood glucose once–twice-weekly, then monthly. Steroid treatment cards should be carried at all times showing Drug/Dose/Duration/Prescriber. Patients who are non-immune should be told to report exposure to chickenpox or measles (may require passive immunization). Bone densitometry is debated. Best considered for those on long-term (> 3months) treatment
Azathioprine/ mercaptopurine	*British National Formulary recommendation*: monitor full blood count weekly for first 4 weeks and at least every 3 months thereafter. Evidence of practical value of this frequency of monitoring is lacking, and less frequent monitoring in inflammatory bowel diseases (full blood count at 2–4 weeks, then every 2–3 months) has been safe in large (n > 600) patient groups.
Methotrexate	Prior to commencement: counselling about pregnancy; measure renal function/liver function tests/full blood count *British National Formulary recommendation*: full blood count and liver function tests weekly for 4 weeks, monthly thereafter. Evidence of practical value of this frequency of monitoring is lacking. *In case of neutropenia*: advise immediate withdrawal (white blood cells < 2.0 x 10^9/l), or dose reduction (white blood cells 2.0–3.5 x 10^9/l). *In case of cough/dyspnoea*: advise chest x-ray and pulmonary function tests. Abnormal liver function tests: advise immediate withdrawal, but may recommence if return to normal. Avoid NSAIDs/aspirin during therapy/penicillins (reduce renal excretion). No conception for 6 months after treatment discontinued (male and female).

Summary of monitoring advice for drugs used in inflammatory bowel disease

Ciclosporin	Drug interactions: calcium antagonists increase ciclosporin concentrations, anti-epileptics decrease its concentrations. For oral ciclosporin: weekly to bi-monthly blood pressure, creatinine and ciclosporin concentration.
Infliximab	*Before infusion:* chest x-ray and confirmation of previous BCG vaccination: check C-reactive protein and measure Harvey-Bradshaw index of Crohn's activity. If no previous BCG, then perform Heaf test. *During infusion:* pulse/blood pressure/temperature/respiratory rate during infusion over 2 hours. *After infusion:* be aware of risk of serious infection in weeks following infusion. Joint pains and other delayed side effects occasionally occur.

Appendix 3 – Useful websites

www.bsg.org.uk
(British Society of Gastroenterology. UK-based society for
gastroenterologists: promotes education, research and best clinical
practice guidelines for gastrointestinal disease.[160])

www.CCFA.org
(Crohn's and Colitis Foundation of America: American non-profit,
volunteer-driven organisation dedicated to finding the cure for
Crohn's disease and ulcerative colitis. Principally raises money for
research. Also provides information for people with inflammatory
bowel disease.)

www.CICRA.org
(Crohn's in Childhood Research Association: aims to create a wider
understanding of Crohn's Disease and ulcerative colitis as it affects
children and young adults. Provides support for sufferers and their
families, and raises funds to support medical research.)

www.digestivedisorders.org.uk
(Digestive Disorders Foundation: funds research into digestive
disorders, provides information for patients and raises national
awareness of the symptoms of digestive diseases.)

www.EFCCA.org
(European Federation of Crohn's and ulcerative Colitis Associations:
European organization of 20 national IBD patient associations, to
facilitate the exchange of information and promote cross-frontier
activities, including representation to European authorities.)

www.nacc.org.uk
(National Association for Crohn's and Colitis: UK patient-based
organization (30,000 members) providing literature on all aspects of
inflammatory bowel disease and practical support for patients with
ulcerative colitis or Crohn's disease. Principal UK fundraiser for
inflammatory bowel disease research. Has a helpline, advises on
benefits, welfare and counselling.)

www.the-ia.org.uk
(Ileostomy and Internal Pouch Support Group: aims to help people
who have to undergo colectomy and creation of either an ileostomy
or an ileo-anal pouch. Provides information and support to patients
and their families.)

Index

Notes: As inflammatory bowel disease is the subject of this book, all index entries refer to this disease unless otherwise indicated. Page numbers followed by "f" indicate figures; page numbers followed by "t" indicate tables; vs. indicates a comparison or differential diagnosis. This index is in letter-by-letter order, whereby spaces and hyphens in main entries are excluded by the alphabetization process.

Rapid Reference

A major new series of pocketbooks

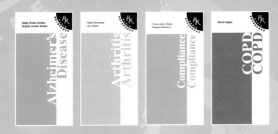
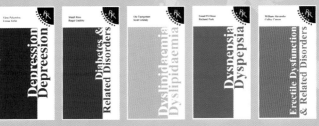
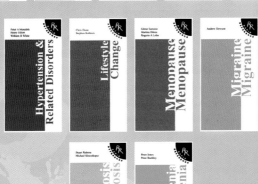

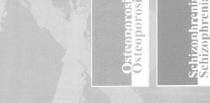

Mosby   www.elsevierhealth.com   ELSEVIER SCIENCE

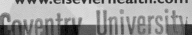